GLOWING UP
RECIPES TO ROCK YOUR NATURAL BEAUTY

Glowing Up: Recipes to Rock Your Natural Beauty is published under Erudition, a sectionalized division under Di Angelo Publications, Inc.

Erudition is an imprint of Di Angelo Publications.
Copyright 2025.
All rights reserved.
Printed in Mexico by Nocaut.

Di Angelo Publications
Los Angeles, California

Library of Congress
Glowing Up: Recipes to Rock Your Natural Beauty
ISBN: 978-1-962603-32-4
Hardback

Words: Carmen & Hilaria Baldwin
Editorial Overview: Alma Felix & Kimberly James
Cover Design: Savina Deianova
Interior Design: Kimberly James
Photography: Victoria Sirakova
Hair and Makeup: Tetiana Kazak
Consulting Dermatologist: Peter L Kopelson, MD
Copyright Attorney: Karen Tripp

Downloadable via www.dapbooks.shop and other e-book retailers.

No part of this publication may be reproduced, distributed, or transmitted in any form or by any means without the prior written permission of the publisher, except in the case of brief quotations embodied in critical reviews and certain other noncommercial uses permitted by copyright law. For permission requests, contact info@diangelopublications.com.

For educational, business, and bulk orders, contact sales@diangelopublications.com.

1. Health & Fitness --- Beauty & Grooming --- Skin Care
2. Juvenile Nonfiction --- Health & Daily Living --- General
3. Crafts & Hobbies --- General

GLOWING UP
RECIPES TO ROCK YOUR NATURAL BEAUTY

Carmen & Hilaria
BALDWIN

CONTENTS

Introduction — 7

Letter from Carmen — 9
Letter from Hilaria — 10

What This Book is About — 12

Let's Get Glowin' — 15
Ingredients — 15
Essential Oils — 16
Supplies — 17
Safe Melting — 18

Recipes — 19

Face — 20
Glow Getter Chia Seed Mask — 21
Glow Boosting Vitamin-C Mask — 22
Nourish & Nurture Carrot & Coconut Mask — 23
Gentle Glow Milky Mask — 24
Kale, Grape, & Cucumber Glow Mask — 25
Oops, Dad's Orange! Turmeric Glow Mask — 26
Tumeric & Yogurt Face Mask — 29
Cool as a Cucumber Face Mask — 30
Oatmeal & Honey Soothing Face Mask — 31
Cocoa & Orange Refreshing Face Mask — 32
Sweet Slumber Night Time Face Mask — 34
Wake Me Up Coffee Scrub — 35
Sweet Dreams Overnight Moisturizer — 36
Banana Blast Face Cleanser — 37
Morning Dew Overnight Face Moisturizer — 38
Hello, Coco! Face Cleanser — 40
Strawbabe Lip Scrub — 41

Cooling Cucumber Lip Mask	42
Glow on the Go Lip Balm	43
Bustling Brows Eyebrow Serum	44

Hair — 46
Go, Go Avocado Hair Mask	47
Rice Water Hair Mask	48
Shiny Hair, I Care! Revitalizing Hair Mask	49
Shake It Out Hair Detangling Spray	50
Scrub Away the Blues Scalp Scrub	51

Body — 52
Silky Smooth Body Scrub	53
Dreamy Feet Foot Mask	54
Nourished Nails Nail & Cuticle Oil	55
Sweet as Honey Milk Bath	56
Tropical Glow Sugar Scrub	57
Banish Those Blues Hydrating Body Oil	58
Sassy Suds Shower Gel	59
Luxuriate Lotion	60

The Secret	62
Let's Talk About Learning to Pamper Yourself	64
Skincare is Self Care	67
Know What's In Your Products	68
Natural Ingredients Around the Globe	70

Glowing Up	74
Let's Skip to the Good Part	76
Safe Place, Safe Space	83
Creativity is Queen	86
Connecting With Her is Key	92
Activities for Mom & Daughter Duos	96
Staying Grounded	100
Mom Tested, Mom Approved	108
Celebrating Mom & Me Around the World	110
Note from the Publisher	112

Safety & Disclaimer

Read this before testing any of the recipes in this book!

None of these recipes are meant as medical advice, and everyone has different skin types, so make sure you are not allergic to anything in the recipes before you put it on your body.

Some of the oils recommended are comedogenic, and some of the ingredients used in the following recipes are potent, so you can adjust the amounts according to your preference.

Every person's skin is different, and as such, may react differently to certain ingredients. Before applying any of the recipes, do a small patch test on your wrist to ensure your skin agrees with it — make sure there is no negative reaction or clogging of the pores.

Be sure to allow the heated ingredients to cool to a safe temperature before handling or applying to skin. When handling anything hot, always make sure an adult is supervising.

The information and perspectives shared in Glowing Up are not intended to diagnose, treat, cure, or prevent any medical condition. Readers should consult a qualified healthcare provider for any health-related concerns or questions.

This book is about having fun as mother and daughter — so don't take it too seriously. Be safe, and enjoy!

INTRODUCTION

Hey everyone!

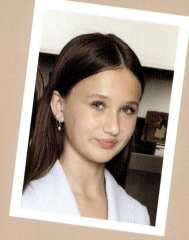

Do you ever feel like you need to look pretty for others — or even for yourself? Maybe it's because some people make you feel like you have to fit into their idea of what "pretty" is. But here's the truth: their opinions don't define you. Pretty isn't one specific thing that someone made up — it's about how you feel inside and out. You are amazing just as you are, and you don't need anyone's approval to be confident every day.

Take care of yourself for you because you deserve it. Self-care isn't about changing who you are; it's about celebrating yourself and feeling your best. I love practicing self-care and sharing it with my mom and friends — it's empowering, and a reminder of how fun it feels to take time for yourself. I hope this book gives you that same feeling.

Skincare and makeup can be fun, creative, and when you use gentle, healthy products, they're great for your skin too. My routine is simple: you can find the ingredients in this book! Healthy ingredients are key — you want to protect your beautiful skin and not cover it up with harsh chemicals!

If you're just starting out, focus on the basics and start with a small routine. The goal is to experiment in a way that feels fun and empowering while embracing your natural beauty. Always remember that you need to make sure you aren't allergic to any of the ingredients. Patch test and always check with your parents. Some of my siblings have allergies and we learn in the house that each one of us can use different things. This should be fun and safe, so start with ingredients that work for you. The best part is that there is always a way to customize each recipe.

To the moms reading this:
• If you're on the fence, don't worry — skincare is safe when done right, and it can help kids be creative and express themselves. It is just face art; it doesn't change who your kids are!
• If you're a mom who already encourages your kids to explore while teaching them to feel comfortable in their own skin, thank you. That balance makes all the difference.

These recipes and tips aren't just about feeling great — they're so fun to do with your family and friends while giving you the tools to celebrate your unique self.

Finally, the most important thing is to stay confident. If someone tries to bring you down, remember this: by not reacting, you've already won. Let them get stuck in their negativity while you rise above it. You are perfect, just as you are, and this book is here to help you embrace you.

Never forget that you are amazing. I hope you have as much fun with these recipes as I do.

Carmen

dear mother,

If your home is like ours, skincare, makeup, and Sephora crazes are part of your children's daily routines and interests. I often find myself trying to balance allowing Carmen to express herself and explore how she wants to present herself to the world, while fostering her understanding that true beauty comes from within. At the same time, I want to protect her from the harsh chemicals found in some of the products she's eager to try, while allowing her to belong amongst her peers and try things out. It's a struggle and a juggle!

The tween years are funny — they're still so young, yet they're starting to step into the woman space. Some people chastise me for letting Carmen wear makeup, but I know I'm not alone in having a daughter who wants to experiment with skincare and makeup. We all went through our own versions of this growing up. We remember those awkward phases: perms or straighteners, jet-black hair, dark lip liner, white lipstick, or slicked-back hair with two strands framing our faces. It's a cycle that repeats across generations with their own versions, a rite of self-discovery, of learning what makes us feel like us, that has become ingrained in the woman experience.

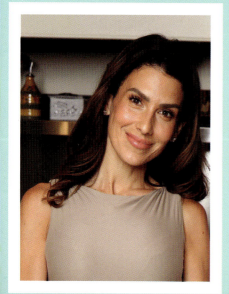

For many, it starts innocently enough — dressing up as a Disney princess, doing face paint, or playing with pretend makeup. That's how it started with Carmen too. It starts to become a "thing" when our daughters begin taking steps into womanhood. The fear of our girls growing up too fast is sparked, as well as the need to protect them from those who might harm them. We may fear that the makeup almost acts like a target, used by others as a reflection of having poor values and beliefs. It's a parent's duty to protect our children from this, and to make sure that we teach them what's truly important.

So, how do we allow our little tweens to express themselves while protecting them from the products and pressures that concern us? Most importantly, how do we help them understand that while skincare and makeup can be fun, true worth and beauty grow from the inside out?

With Carmen, I try to separate the idea of skincare and makeup from the concept of beauty. She's inevitably exposed to social media, filters, and peer pressure, but I hope that by focusing on and nurturing the beauty in her soul, she'll learn this distinction for herself. I want her to see makeup and skincare as fun ways to express herself, not as a mask to hide behind. If her inner self-confidence is strong, skincare and makeup become tools for play and creativity. And you can take them or leave them.

Allowing Carmen to pamper herself and take the time for self-care is something I hope she will carry with her throughout her life, in whatever way feels authentic to her. Teaching her that she deserves "me time," and that not everything worth pampering herself with needs to be a colorful product, packaged and promoted by an influencer. It's more about what feels right and can be mixed with the same ingredients she would put inside her body. Does this mean she doesn't buy makeup from the store and play with this too? Of course she does . . . but it is part of the balance to expose her to the understanding that there is more than one way, and most importantly: there is no ONE right way. Sometimes these hints and lessons we slip in will sink in deeply enough and form a strong foundation for her future.

One way we explore this balance is through DIY skincare. In our home, we see these recipes as a steppingstone from the mud, sand, and leaf pies Carmen would once make in the park, mix with a stick, and pretend to feed me with. The recipes in this book are made from whole ingredients that can go from the supermarket to the pantry, to their faces. Please make sure that your kids aren't allergic to any of the ingredients. Some of my kids have allergies and we must always be aware of what works for each one. I have learned that oils, dairy, nuts, and other ingredients can create sensitivity in some people. So just take care; these should be fun activities that are safe for all. There are always ways to customize each recipe to make sure it is safe. Also, there are places that ask for safe melting or heating of certain ingredients; make sure that they are always supervised and helped with anything that involves heat and that proper cooling is practiced. There are points where the blender is used as well. Just look out to make sure that your child is being safe!

Much of this book was Carmen-driven. Watching her research and experiment with different masks and scrubs was so much fun. She would mix her concoctions, disappear for a while, and then reappear with a face mask on, proudly explaining the benefits of each ingredient. Her strawberry lip scrub is my favorite — I ask her to make it for me all the time.

So, have fun and mix away with your little ones! I hope you find these activities not only enjoyable but also empowering and meaningful — a chance to bond while nurturing self-care and self-expression.

hilaria

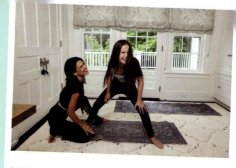

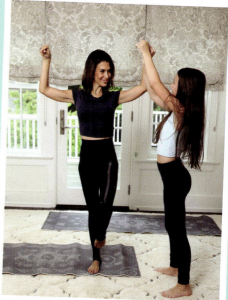

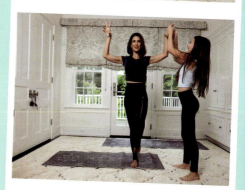

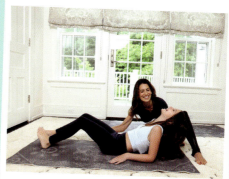

Q & A

Q: What is the book about? How would you describe it?

Carmen: I am sharing my skincare and skin-related recipes that I have fun playing with and pampering myself with. It's also about having fun experimenting with my family, my friends, or just by myself, especially if I'm bored! I've been making my own skincare for a while — taking things from the kitchen and trying them out, like coffee scrubs or rice masks. I like figuring out how different ingredients work together, learning about measurements and consistency. It's like science, but you get to put it on your face!

Q: Why do you want to make this book? Why is it important to you?

Carmen: I just love experimenting, honestly. The other day, I made a rice mask with milk, honey, and herbs from a teabag. My mom has tried to bring me to a spa before, but they said I was too young, so I decided to just do it myself in my home! I want other kids my age to be able to have fun like this, so I wanted to write this book to share. I also know a lot of people are scared of what's in their products. This book shows you that you can make it yourself and it's safe!

Q: What do you want readers to take away from your book?

Carmen: I want people to realize that skincare can be easy and fun. Like, you don't need to spend on products we see people trying to sell us when you can make a cool mask with stuff you already have. I want readers to feel proud because they did it themselves. Most importantly, there can be so much pressure to focus on looking a certain way, and I want this book to feel like an invitation to celebrate yourself without trying to conform to anything or anyone.

Our mothers are usually our first role models. Moms dream of their daughters growing up to be confident and successful, and they also set examples by the way they care for themselves. This "taking care" can be anything, but it has to feel good and self-nurturing. Mothers are often shamed for taking "me time." Teaching our children that taking care of ourselves is well deserved and it also gives them the roadmap that one day, they too may be parents, and they are just as worthy of always being human.

Skincare can be fun and creative, a way to play with self-expression. But as a tween, skin is still changing, and some products out there — like anti-aging creams — aren't meant for children and could actually harm the skin.

This book explores how to embrace yourself and make smart choices when it comes to skincare and makeup. Instead of following quickly evolving trends that aren't meant for young skin, our children can learn how to choose safe, natural products that help them feel their best. It's not about hiding or changing but rather pampering themselves and feeling good and authentic!

In this book, you'll also find parenting ideas we try at home, about growing up, navigating changes, and building self-confidence. Whether it's learning how to care for skin, finding personal style, or understanding that beauty comes from being authentic, this book is intended to be an inspiration to feeling good inside and out.

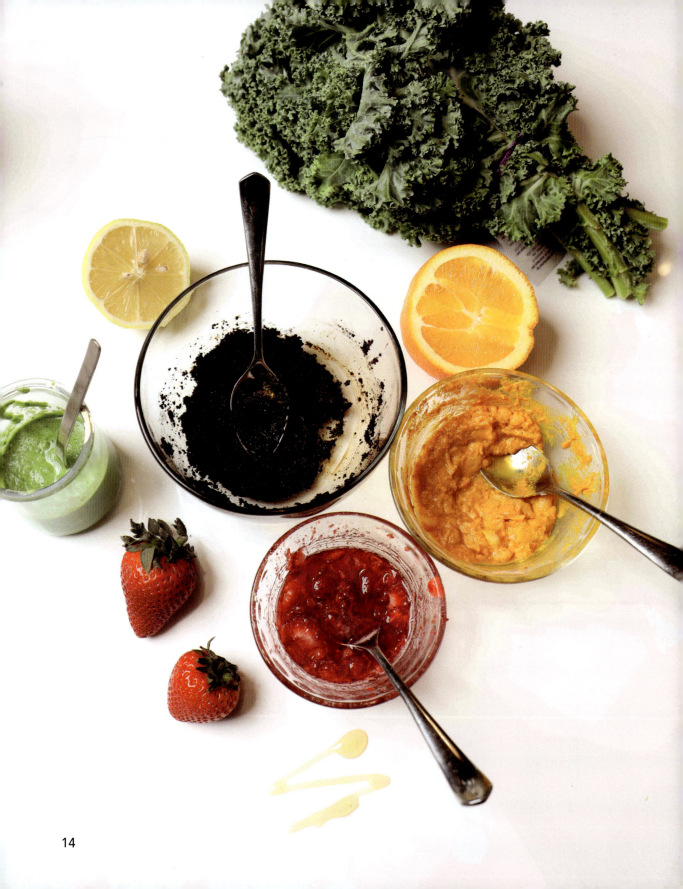

LET'S GET GLOWIN'

EVERYTHING YOU NEED TO START PUTTING TOGETHER YOUR GLOW

INGREDIENTS

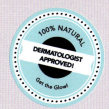

The ingredients in the following recipes are natural (nat•u•ral) – commonly found in nature, and not humanmade. Your kitchen and local grocery store are treasure troves for natural ingredients. Everyday items like honey, yogurt, avocado, and oats can be transformed into soothing face masks or nourishing scrubs. A stroll through the produce aisle might inspire a DIY glow serum with cucumber or a gentle exfoliant with fresh lemon and sugar. Even pantry staples like coconut oil or chia seeds can work wonders for your skin. The best part? These ingredients are affordable and free of the harsh chemicals found in many store-bought products. It's like creating a mini spa experience right at home, using nature's finest!

Here are some of the more common ingredients you'll find throughout this book. The list gives a bit of a behind-the-scenes peek at how these superfoods can work for you!

- **Aloe:** Known for its soothing and hydrating properties, aloe vera helps calm irritated skin, reduces redness, and provides moisture without feeling greasy.

- **Beeswax:** A natural barrier that locks in moisture, beeswax protects the skin from environmental irritants while keeping it soft and hydrated.

- **Coconut Oil:** Rich in fatty acids, coconut oil deeply moisturizes the skin, helps reduce dryness, and has antimicrobial properties that can help with minor skin irritations.

- **Honey:** A natural humectant, honey attracts and retains moisture in the skin. It also has antibacterial properties and can promote healing for blemishes.

- **Turmeric:** Packed with antioxidants and anti-inflammatory compounds, turmeric brightens the skin, reduces redness, and helps even out skin tone.

- **Yogurt:** The lactic acid in yogurt gently exfoliates the skin, removing dead cells and leaving it smooth and glowing. It also soothes and nourishes the skin with its probiotics.

- **Avocado:** Rich in vitamins and healthy fats, avocado deeply hydrates and nourishes the skin, promoting elasticity and a radiant glow.

- **Sugar:** A natural exfoliant, sugar removes dead skin cells and smooths the skin, leaving it soft and refreshed.

- **Milk:** The lactic acid in milk gently exfoliates while its fats and proteins hydrate and soften the skin, giving it a healthy, supple appearance.

- **Chia Seeds:** Loaded with omega-3 fatty acids and antioxidants, chia seeds help hydrate the skin, reduce inflammation, and protect it from environmental damage.

ESSENTIAL OILS

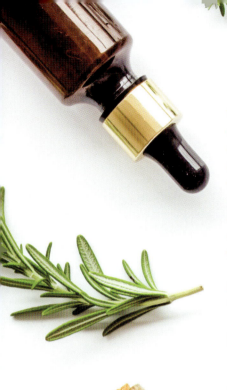

Some recipes in this book call for the addition of a few drops of essential oils. Because they smell great, essential oils can be wonderful additions to your beauty routine, but they should be used carefully and responsibly to avoid irritation or damage. Before selecting an oil, check with an adult to make sure it is safe to use on skin. And just because "essential" is in the name, it doesn't mean the oil is essential to the recipe. If you are allergic or sensitive to oils, the recipes work just fine without them! The scents are nice to add but not at all necessary.

Five Common Essential Oils and Their Benefits:
1. **Lavender:** Known for its calming scent, lavender essential oil helps soothe irritated skin, reduce redness, and promote relaxation.
2. **Tea Tree:** A popular choice for acne-prone skin, tea tree oil has strong antibacterial and antifungal properties that help combat breakouts and soothe inflammation.
3. **Rosemary:** This oil improves circulation and promotes healthy, glowing skin. It's often used in hair care to stimulate growth and reduce dandruff.
4. **Chamomile:** Gentle and soothing, chamomile essential oil reduces redness and irritation, making it ideal for sensitive or inflamed skin.
5. **Lemon:** Rich in vitamin C, lemon essential oil helps brighten skin, even out tone, and reduce oiliness. It's also used to exfoliate and refresh the skin.

What to Know About Using Essential Oils in Skincare:
6. **Dilution is Key:** Essential oils are highly concentrated and should never be applied directly to the skin. Always dilute them with a carrier oil (like coconut, jojoba, or almond oil) before use.
7. **Patch Test First:** Before using an essential oil, do a patch test on a small area of skin to ensure you don't have an allergic reaction or sensitivity.
8. **Avoid Sensitive Areas:** Keep essential oils away from sensitive areas like the eyes, mouth, and open wounds, as they can cause irritation or harm.
9. **Sun Sensitivity:** Some oils, like lemon and other citrus oils, can make your skin more sensitive to sunlight. Avoid using them on exposed skin if you'll be in the sun.
10. **Quality Matters:** Always choose high-quality, pure essential oils from reputable sources. Avoid synthetic or adulterated oils, which can be harmful to the skin.

SUPPLIES

You'll want to gather these supplies before you start whipping up your creations:
- Measuring cups
- Mixing bowls
- Spoon
- Knife
- Whisk
- Funnel
- Blender or hand mixer
- Double boiler
- Molds

It's important to use new and clean containers to store your products in to keep them fresh and prevent mold from growing. You can find many of these items at grocery stores, drug stores, craft stores, or online.
- Glass jars
- Spray Bottles
- Squeeze Bottles
- Spice tins or jars
- Screw top containers
- Lockets
- Mint tin
- Cotton swabs
- Disposable mascara wands

Once your creations are complete, store them in a cool, dry place. Never use a product if it looks like it has grown mold, changed colors, or smells bad.

If you have skin sensitivites or allergies, please check with your doctor or dermatologist before using any of these recipes.

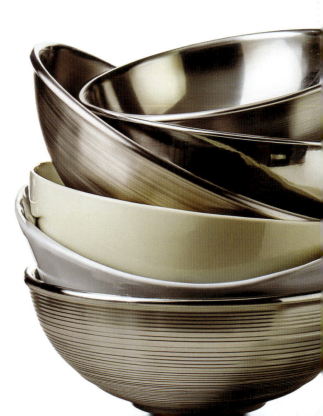

SAFE MELTING
(ADULT SUPERVISION NEEDED)

Some ingredients, like coconut oil and shea butter, are usually stored as solids, but to make these recipes, you will need to melt them.

You can use a microwave to do this by heating the product in 30-second increments at 50% power until melted. Be sure to use a microwave-safe container when heating, and wear oven mitts when removing hot objects from the microwave to avoid burning yourself.

Be sure to allow the heated ingredients to cool to a safe temperature before handling or applying to skin. When handling anything hot, always make sure an adult is supervising!

Another melting method involves a double boiler. Using a double boiler at home is simple and an excellent way to gently heat or melt ingredients without direct contact with intense heat. Here's how to do it:

What You'll Need:
- A medium to large pot
- A heatproof bowl (glass or metal) that fits snugly over the pot but doesn't touch the water
- The ingredients you want to heat or melt

Steps to Use a Double Boiler:
1. **Fill the Pot with Water:** Add about 1–2 inches of water to the pot. The water level should be low enough that it won't touch the bottom of the heatproof bowl when placed on top.
2. **Heat the Water:** Place the pot on the stove and heat the water over medium to low heat until it starts to simmer gently. Avoid boiling the water, as the steam is what will heat the bowl.
3. **Set the Bowl on the Pot:** Place the heatproof bowl on top of the pot. It should sit securely without tipping or letting steam escape from the sides.
4. **Add Your Ingredients:** Put the ingredients you want to heat or melt into the bowl.
5. **Stir Gently:** Use a heatproof spatula or spoon to stir the ingredients gently and continuously for even heating.
6. **Monitor the Heat:** Keep an eye on the water to ensure it stays at a simmer. If it starts to boil, reduce the heat to prevent the bowl from getting too hot.
7. **Remove When Done:** Once the ingredients are fully melted or heated, carefully lift the bowl off the pot using oven mitts or a towel, as it will be hot.
8. **Turn Off the Stove:** Turn off the stove and allow the pot to cool before handling or cleaning.

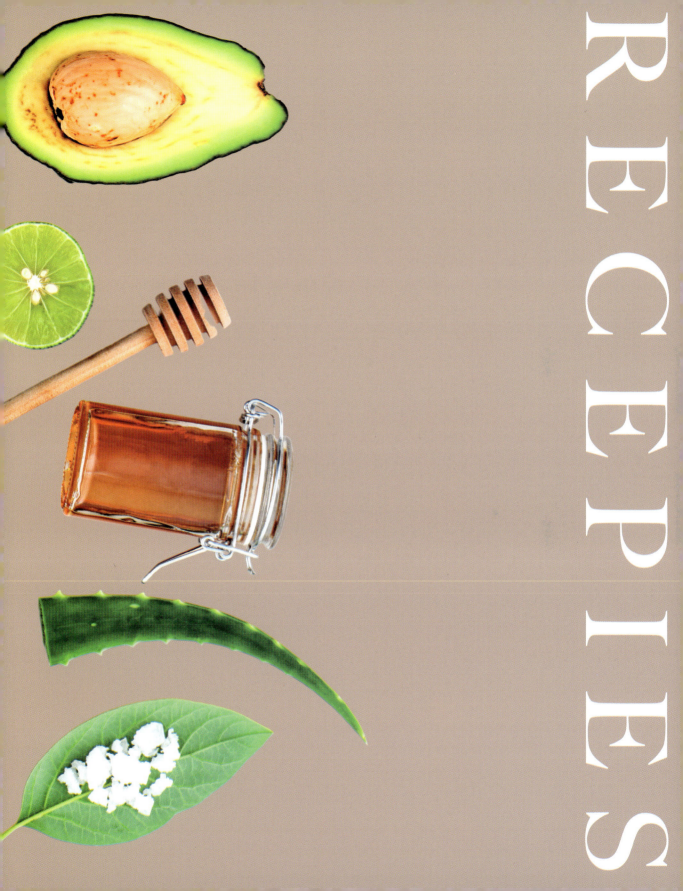

RECEPIES

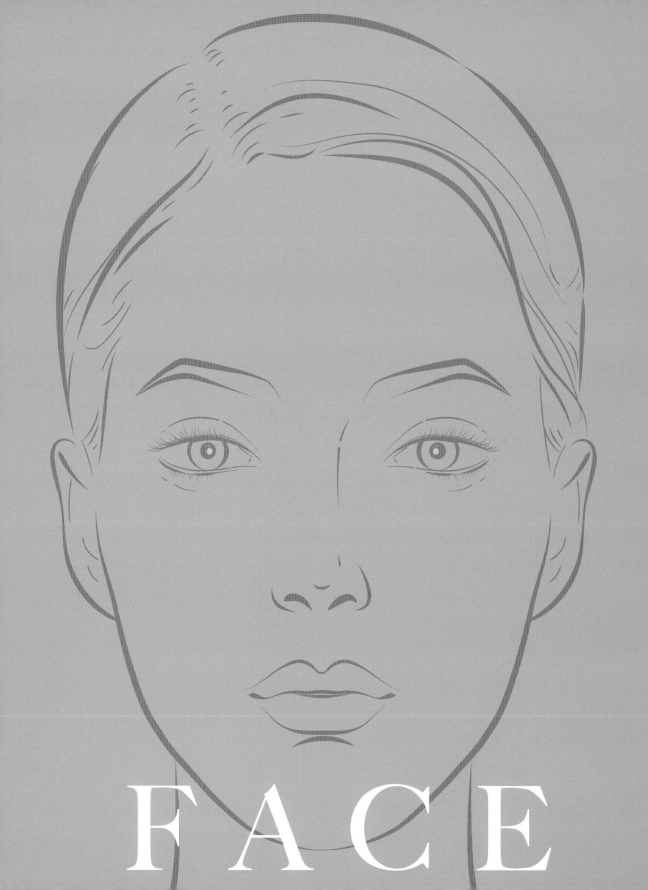

GLOW GETTER
CHIA SEED MASK

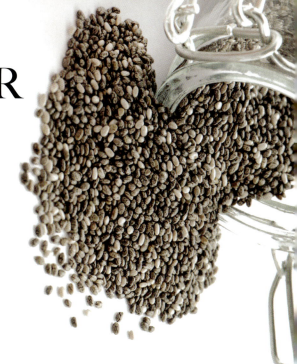

Get ready to pamper your skin with a mask as nourishing as it is simple! This DIY Glow Getter Chia Seed Mask combines the natural hydration of chia seeds, the soothing touch of honey, and the pure magic of water. Perfect for giving your skin a radiant boost, this mask is like a hug for your face — gentle, revitalizing, and oh-so-refreshing. This simple, natural mask is your secret weapon for radiant skin!

INGREDIENTS

- 2 tbsp chia seeds
- 1 cup water
- 1 tsp honey

MAKE IT

1. Mix chia seeds and water in a bowl. Let it sit for 10 minutes, and watch in amazement as the seeds transform into a magical gel!

2. Stir in that golden goodness - honey! It's nature's moisturizer, adding a touch of sweetness to your skin.

3. Apply the gel to your face, avoiding the eye area. Relax for 10 minutes, letting the mask work its hydrating magic.

4. Rinse off the mask with warm water and follow up with your favorite cleanser.

YOU GLOW, GIRL!

Now it's time to reveal your glow! Voila! Your skin will feel refreshed, hydrated, and ready to shine!

GLOW BOOSTING
VITAMIN-C MASK

Vitamins for your skin! This glow boosting Vitamin C mask is packed with the natural goodness of fresh orange juice and gentle exfoliating powder of baking soda. This mask will leave your skin feeling hydrated, smooth and refreshed. Perfect for a quick pick-me-up, it's an easy, all natural way to add a radiant glow to your day!

INGREDIENTS

- 2 tbsp fresh orange juice
- 1 tsp baking soda

MAKE IT

1. In a small bowl, combine the orange juice and baking soda. The mixture will fizz slightly as the ingredients react — that's normal! Stir until fully blended.
2. Using clean fingers or a brush, apply the mask evenly to your face, avoiding the eyes and mouth.
3. Leave the mask on for 2–5 minutes. You may feel a slight tingling sensation — this is the mask working its magic!
4. Rinse off with lukewarm water, gently massaging in circular motions for extra exfoliation. Pat dry and follow with your favorite moisturizer.

YOU GLOW, GIRL!

Vitamin C is great for the skin, and baking soda is a gentle exfoliant.

Use this mask 1–2 times per week for best results. Always do a patch test before using new ingredients on your skin to check for sensitivity. Remember that oranges are acidic, so if the tingling sensation is too intense, go ahead and wash off the mask. For extra hydration, add 1 tsp of honey or aloe vera gel to the mixture.

Get ready to glow with a fresh, bright complexion, courtesy of this Vitamin C treat!

NOURISH & NURTURE
CARROT & COCONUT MASK

Give your skin a dose of natural goodness with this Nourishing Carrot & Coconut Mask! Carrots, packed with beta-carotene and antioxidants, work to take care of your skin, while coconut's deep hydration leaves it feeling soft, smooth, and radiant. This mask is a perfect way to refresh and nourish your complexion. Feel the nourishing power of carrots and coconuts transform your skin into a glowing, hydrated masterpiece!

INGREDIENTS

- 2 tbsp carrot puree
- 1 tbsp coconut oil (if allergic, substitue your favorite oil)
- 1 tsp honey

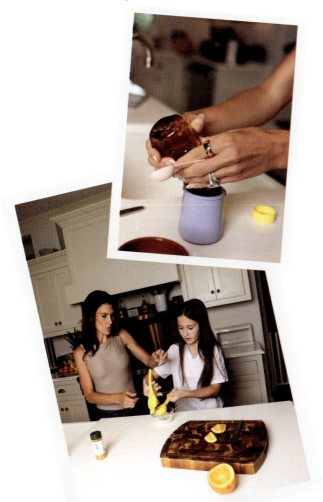

MAKE IT

1. Steam or boil a small carrot until soft (always have adult supervision when handling hot ingredients), then mash it into a smooth puree. Allow it to cool to room temperature.

2. In a bowl, combine the carrot puree, coconut oil, and honey. Stir until the ingredients are well blended.

3. Using clean fingers or a brush, apply the mask evenly to your face, avoiding the eyes and mouth.

4. Leave the mask on for 5–10 minutes. Use this time to unwind and let your skin soak up the nutrients.

5. Rinse off with lukewarm water, gently massaging your skin to boost circulation. Pat dry and follow with your favorite moisturizer.

YOU GLOW, GIRL!

Use this mask once a week for a natural glow. For an extra cooling effect, store the mask in the fridge for 10 minutes before applying. Always do a patch test to ensure your skin loves the natural ingredients.

GENTLE GLOW
MILKY MASK

Treat your skin to a soothing and hydrating experience with this Gentle Glow Milky Mask! Combining the moisturizing and exfoliating properties of milk with the antibacterial and nourishing benefits of honey, this simple mask is perfect for giving your skin a natural glow. It's a quick, all-natural way to pamper yourself. Indulge in this creamy, dreamy mask and enjoy the radiant, silky-smooth skin it leaves behind!

INGREDIENTS

- 2 tbsp milk (or your fave milk alternative)
- 1 tbsp honey

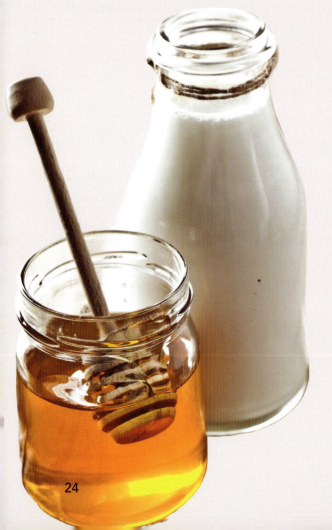

MAKE IT

1. In a small bowl, whisk together the milk and honey until fully combined. The mixture should be smooth and slightly thick.

2. Using a clean brush or your fingertips, apply the mask evenly to your face and neck, avoiding the eye area.

3. Leave the mask on for 10–15 minutes, allowing the ingredients to work their magic.

4. Gently rinse with lukewarm water, massaging your skin in circular motions. Pat your face dry with a clean towel.

5. Follow with your favorite moisturizer to lock in the hydration.

YOU GLOW, GIRL!

Allergic to dairy? No problem! Your favorite dairy-free milk alternative will work just as well. For an added boost, mix in 1 tsp of oat flour for gentle exfoliation. Use once or twice a week to maintain soft, glowing skin. Always use fresh ingredients for the best results.

KALE, GRAPE, & CUCUMBER
GLOW MASK

Get ready to glow! This natural mask is packed with vitamins and antioxidants to nourish your skin.

INGREDIENTS

- 4 grapes
- 1 kale leaf
- 1/8 cup sunflower oil
- 1/2 cucumber

MAKE IT

1. Prep your ingredients. Wash the grapes, kale leaf, and cucumber, thoroughly. Remove the seeds from the grapes. Peel the cucumber.

2. In a blender, combine the grapes, kale leaf, cucumber, and sunflower oil. Blend until you have a smooth paste. Ask an adult for help with this step.

3. Cleanse your face with a gentle cleanser. Apply the mask evenly to your face and neck, avoiding the eye and mouth area. Relax for 15–20 minutes.

4. Rinse the mask off with warm water. Pat your face dry with a soft towel. Apply a moisturizer to lock in hydration.

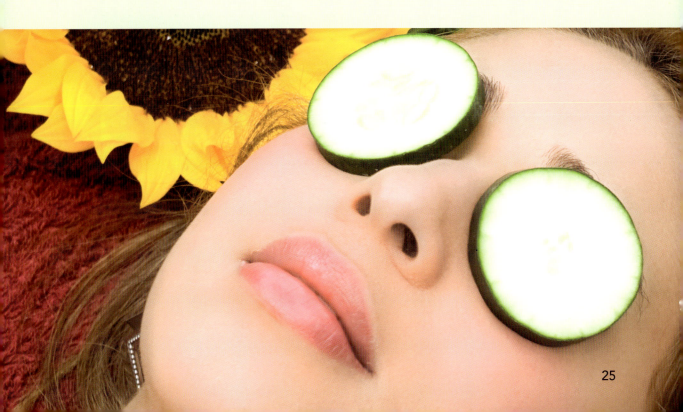

CREATING RECIPES
AND TRYING THEM OUT...

If you're going to try out your recipes on someone other than yourself, make sure your test subject is willing. I like to use my dad, when he's willing (and feeling brave). Mom and I were so excited to try and make our own turmeric face mask. Here's the recipe we came up with:

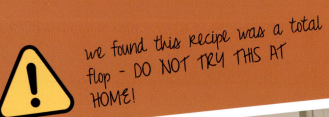

we found this recipe was a total flop - DO NOT TRY THIS AT HOME!

INGREDIENTS
- 1/4 cup virgin coconut oil
- 2 tbsp turmeric powder
- 1 teaspoon sunflower oil
- Juice of 1/3 orange

MAKE IT
1. In a small bowl, combine all the ingredients. Stir until you have a smooth paste.
2. Wash your face with a gentle cleanser to remove dirt and oil.
3. Using clean fingers, apply the mask evenly to your face and neck, avoiding your eyes and lips.
4. Leave the mask on for 15–20 minutes. Relax and let the magic happen!
5. Rinse your face with warm water, gently massaging your skin.
6. Finish with a light moisturizer to lock in hydration.

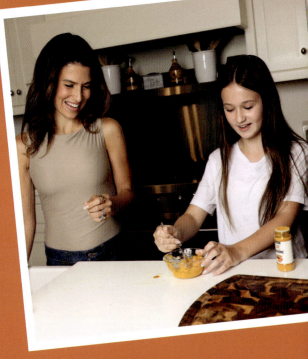

 DO NOT ATTEMPT THIS RECIPE!

testing, testing...

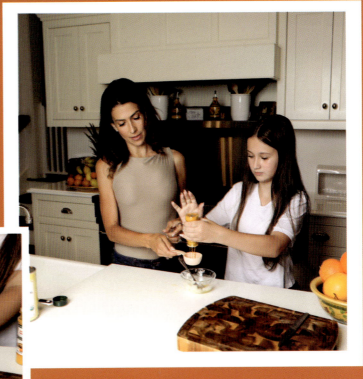

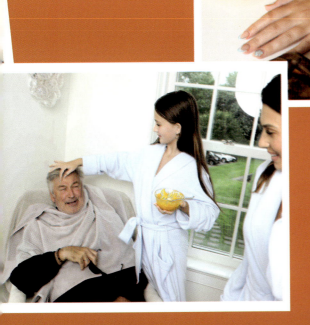

OOPS...

27

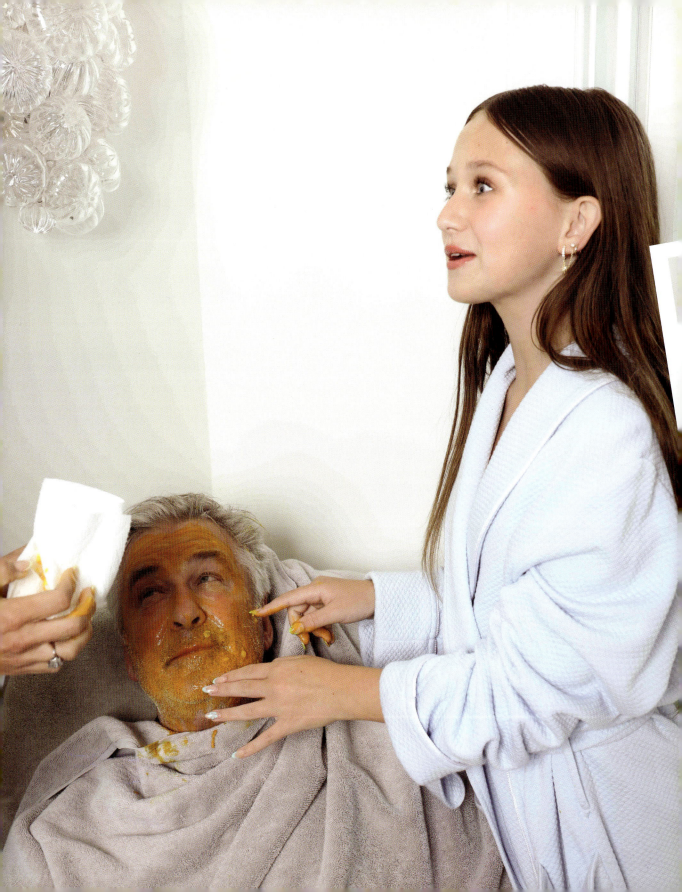

WE TURNED DAD ORANGE!

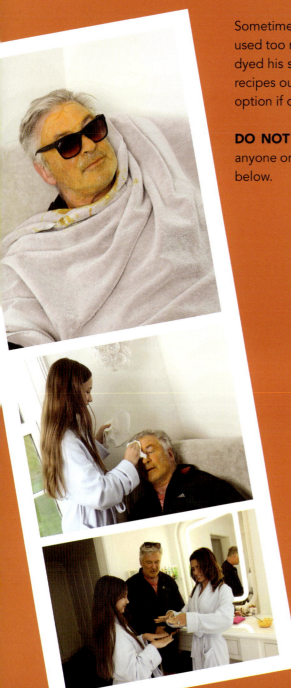

Sometimes, new recipes take a few times to perfect. I think we used too much turmeric, and mixed with citrus juice, it literally dyed his skin — at least for a day. It's always important to test recipes out. I like to use the top of my hand, and that's a great option if dad's not around.

DO NOT try the previous turmeric mask recipe and turn anyone orange! Instead, try this turmeric and yogurt face mask below.

INGREDIENTS
- 1/8 tsp turmeric powder
- 1 tsp argan oil (or your fave oil)
- 2 tbsp plain yogurt (or your fave yogurt alternative)

MAKE IT

1. Mix turmeric powder and argan oil in a small bowl.

2. Gradually add yogurt (or alternative liquid) while stirring to form a smooth paste.

3. Apply the mask evenly to your face. Leave it on for 5 minutes.

4. Gently massage your skin as you rinse the mask off with lukewarm water.

COOL AS A CUCUMBER
FACE MASK

Hey, glow-getters! Want to give your skin a refreshing treat? This Cucumber & Yogurt Face Mask is the ultimate way to chill out while keeping your skin soft and happy. Cucumbers are packed with hydration, and yogurt helps to soothe and smooth — talk about a dream team!

INGREDIENTS
- 1 cold cucumber, peeled
- 1/2 cup yogurt (dairy or non-dairy if needed!)

MAKE IT
1. Blend the cucumber until it's smooth and juicy. Have an adult help you with this step.
2. Stir in the yogurt until it's a creamy, dreamy mixture.
3. Apply to your face (avoiding your eyes) and let it sit for 5 minutes.
4. Rinse off with cool water and pat dry.

YOU GLOW, GIRL!
Now, enjoy your fresh, glowing skin! Keep this in the fridge for extra chill vibes! Add 1 teaspoon of honey for extra moisture and glow — honey is nature's little skin superhero! Blend in a spoonful of mashed avocado for deep hydration and that dewy goddess look! Put on your favorite playlist, grab some cucumber slices for your eyes, and relax like the self-care queen you are!

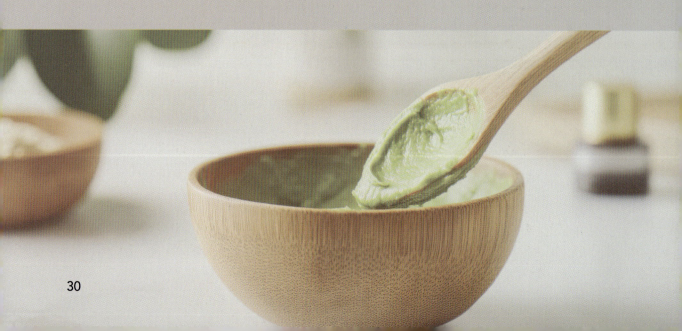

OATMEAL & HONEY
SOOTHING FACE MASK

This Oatmeal & Honey Face Mask is like a cozy blanket for your skin! It's super easy to make, gentle on skin, and uses stuff you probably already have in your kitchen. Say hello to smooth, glowing skin. Plus, it's totally fun to mix up your own spa day potion — perfect for a solo pampering sesh or a sleepover activity with friends!

INGREDIENTS
- 2 tbsp finely ground oats or oat flour
- 1 tbsp honey
- 1–2 tbsp warm water or chamomile tea

MAKE IT
1. If you don't have oat flour, blend oats in a food processor until they're super fine. Have an adult help you with this step.
2. In a small bowl, combine the ground oats, honey, and 1 tablespoon of warm water or chamomile tea. Add more liquid a little at a time until you have a smooth, spreadable paste.
3. Apply the mixture to your clean, dry face in gentle, circular motions. Avoid your eyes and mouth.
4. Leave the mask on for 5–10 minutes while you relax.
5. Wash off the mask with warm water, gently massaging your skin as you go. Pat dry and admire that glow!

YOU GLOW, GIRL!

Your skin is thanking you for all that oatmeal goodness (soothing and softening) and honey magic (hydrating and antibacterial). Whether you're getting ready for a fun day or winding down, this mask is the perfect way to show your skin some love. So go rock your glow and remember — you're absolutely fabulous, just the way you are!

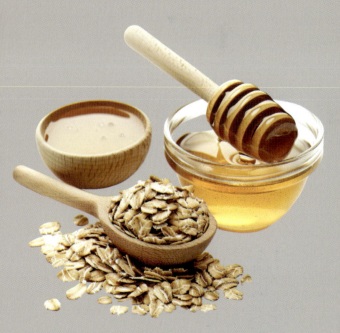

COCOA & ORANGE
REFRESHING FACE MASK

You're about to whip up a chocolatey face mask that smells just as good as it feels! This Cocoa & Orange Mask is like a dessert for your skin — hydrating, brightening, and totally fun to make. Plus, with ingredients like cocoa powder and orange zest, you'll feel like a skincare chef in no time. Ready to treat your face to a spa moment that's as sweet as you are? Let's do this!

INGREDIENTS
- 1 tbsp unsweetened cocoa powder
- 1 tbsp plain yogurt or mashed avocado
- 1/2 tsp orange zest from a fresh orange
- 1 tsp honey

YOU GLOW, GIRL!
This mask not only smells incredible but also leaves your skin feeling fresh, soft, and oh-so-glowy. Keep this recipe handy for whenever you need a quick pick-me-up or a fun DIY with your mom or your besties.

MAKE IT
1. Use a fine grater or zester to get a pinch of fresh orange zest. Ask an adult for help with this part. Be careful to only scrape the orange part — no bitter white bits!
2. In a small bowl, combine the cocoa powder, yogurt (or avocado), orange zest, and honey. Stir until it forms a smooth, creamy paste.
3. Gently spread the mask over your clean, dry face, avoiding your eyes and mouth.
4. Let the mask sit for 5–10 minutes.
5. Wash the mask off with warm water, massaging gently as you go. Pat your skin dry and prepare to be amazed!

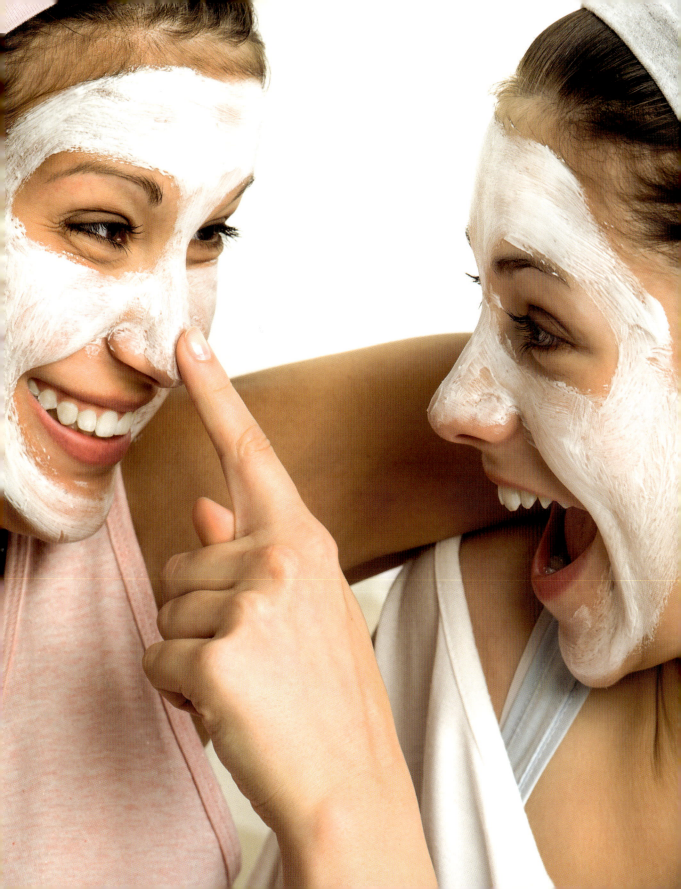

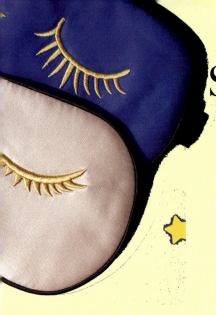

SWEET SLUMBER
NIGHT TIME FACE MASK

This rich, nourishing mask is perfect for right before going to sleep, soaking your skin in deep hydration. Infused with soothing ingredients that calm and refresh, it melts into your skin, so you wake up with a soft, radiant glow — like you just had the sweetest beauty sleep!

INGREDIENTS

- 1/2 ripe avocado
- 1 tbsp rice powder
- 2 tbsp milk (or fave dairy-free alternative)
- 1 tsp honey

MAKE IT

1. In a bowl, mash the avocado until smooth and creamy, free of lumps.
2. Stir in the rice powder.
3. Add the milk and stir until well combined.
4. Mix in the honey.
5. Stir everything together until you have a smooth, thick paste.

YOU GLOW, GIRL!

After cleansing your face in the evening, apply the mask evenly to your skin. Let it sit for 5–10 minutes to absorb. Rinse off with lukewarm water before bed.

WAKE ME UP
COFFEE SCRUB

Packed with energizing coffee grounds and nourishing oils, Wake Me Up Scrub has a magical power to exfoliate and reveal a glowing, refreshed complexion. With a burst of excitement, it goes to work, gently exfoliating while the rich aroma of coffee dances in the air. With every scrub, it leaves skin feeling soft, revitalized, and ready to take on the day!

INGREDIENTS

- 1/4 cup used coffee grounds
- 1 tbsp honey
- 1/8 cup water
- 1/8 tsp turmeric

MAKE IT

1. Combine into a small bowl.
2. Stir to thoroughly mix into a scrub.
3. Gently scrub the mixture onto your face or body.
4. Rinse off with water.

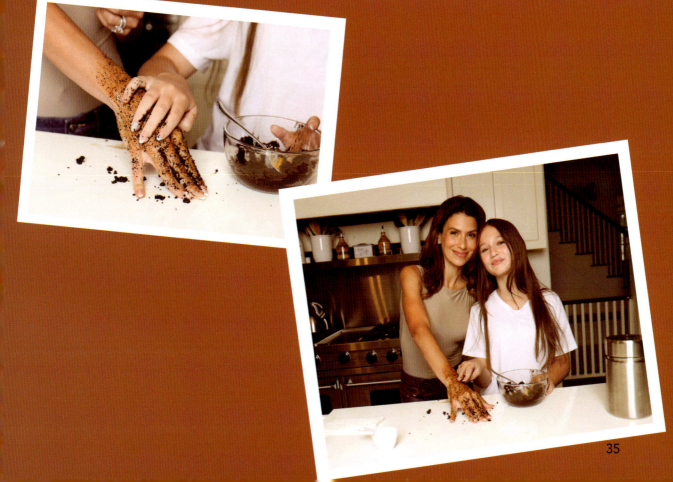

SWEET DREAMS
OVERNIGHT MOISTURIZER

This rich, calming blend will leave your skin feeling soft and supple by morning! With deeply hydrating shea butter, moisturizing coconut oil, and an optional hint of lavender essential oil (or whatever essential oil works for your skin), this moisturizer is like a luxurious bedtime treat for your skin. Perfect for dry skin, this formula works its magic overnight to help you wake up with a radiant, well-rested glow.

INGREDIENTS

- 1 tbsp shea butter
- 1 tbsp coconut oil (or your favorite alternative oil)
- (optional) 1 drop lavender essential oil

MAKE IT

1. In a small, clean container, combine the shea butter and coconut oil. Stir or gently melt the mixture if needed, until smooth and creamy. Add the lavender oil and mix well.
2. Before bed, cleanse your skin, then take a small amount of the moisturizer and gently massage it onto your skin.
3. Leave the moisturizer on overnight to allow the rich oils to nourish your skin as you sleep.

YOU GLOW, GIRL!

Use a few nights a week or whenever your skin needs extra hydration. Wake up with soft, smooth, and beautifully moisturized skin!

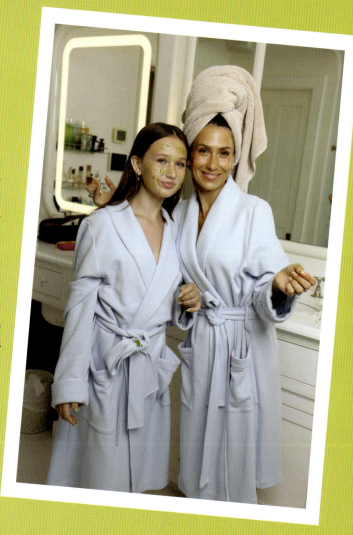

BANANA BLAST
FACE CLEANSER

This delightful blend of creamy banana, lemon, and zingy apple cider vinegar is here to give your face a fresh, radiant glow! Think of it as a smoothie for your skin – gentle, natural, and packed with ingredients to leave you feeling soft, smooth, and oh-so-squeaky clean. Perfect for a little self-care treat, this cleanser is ready to brighten up your routine and give you that just-washed glow. So go on, give your skin the fruity hug it deserves!

INGREDIENTS

- 1 ripe banana, mashed
- 1/8 tsp fresh lemon juice
- 1/8 tsp apple cider vinegar
- 1 tbsp coconut oil (or your fave alternative oil)

MAKE IT

1. In a small bowl, mash the banana until smooth, then stir in the lemon juice, apple cider vinegar, and coconut oil. Mix it all together like you're making a magical skin smoothie!

2. Gently massage this sweet mixture onto your face in little circles. Imagine you're giving yourself a mini spa treatment! Be careful around your eyes and mouth.

3. Rinse off with warm water, pat dry with a soft towel, and say hello to your fresh, radiant skin!

YOU GLOW, GIRL!

Meet your skin's new fruity BFF! Enjoy this treat once or twice a week for a bright and happy complexion! Remember that some of these ingredients have acidic qualities, so if it tingles too intensely, go ahead and wash off the mask.

MORNING DEW
OVERNIGHT FACE MOISTURIZER

While you dream, this luxurious cream works its magic, deeply hydrating and nourishing your skin, so you can rise and shine with a radiant, refreshed complexion. Infused with rich, natural ingredients, it melts into your skin overnight, locking in moisture and smoothing away the day's stress. By morning, you'll be greeted with soft, supple skin that feels as fresh as the first drop of morning dew. Ready to glow? This overnight wonder has you covered!

INGREDIENTS
- 2 tbsp shea butter
- 1 tbsp coconut oil (or your fave alternative oil)

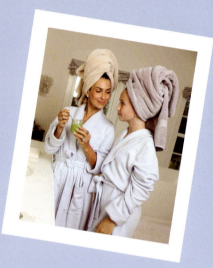

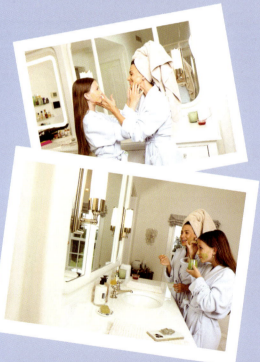

MAKE IT
1. In the microwave, in short intervals, gently melt the shea butter and coconut oil together until fully liquid. (Ask an adult for help with this step.)
2. Let the mixture cool, but don't let it solidify yet.
3. For a light, fluffy texture, you can whip the mixture using a small whisk or hand mixer until it becomes creamy,
4. Pour the moisturizer into a small, clean jar and let it solidify at room temperature or in the fridge.

YOU GLOW, GIRL!

After cleansing your face in the evening, take a small amount of the moisturizer and gently massage it into your skin. Focus on dry areas, and allow the rich oils to absorb overnight. Be careful not to get the moisturizer in your eyes! Wake up with soft, deeply hydrated skin!

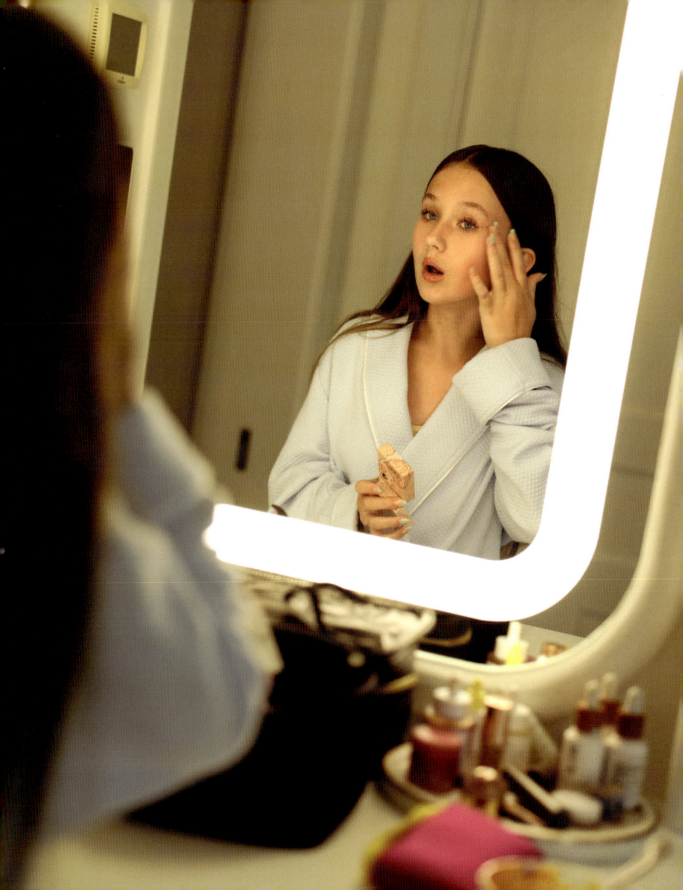

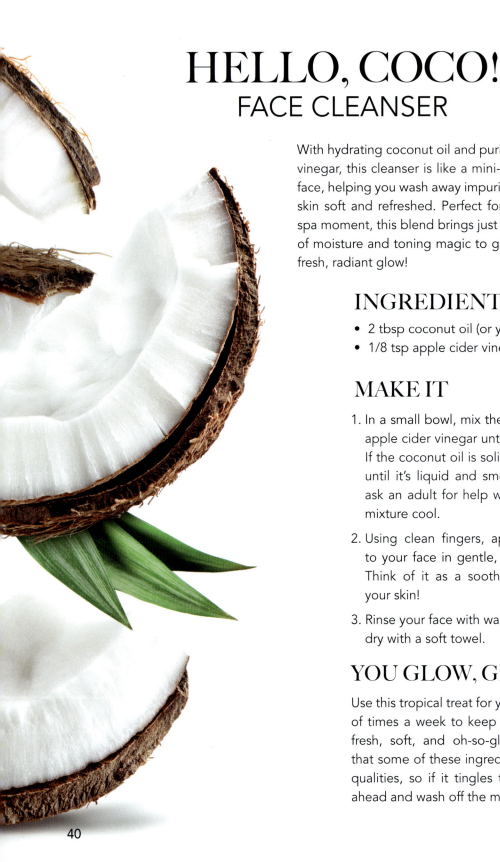

HELLO, COCO!
FACE CLEANSER

With hydrating coconut oil and purifying apple cider vinegar, this cleanser is like a mini-vacation for your face, helping you wash away impurities while leaving skin soft and refreshed. Perfect for a little at-home spa moment, this blend brings just the right balance of moisture and toning magic to give your skin that fresh, radiant glow!

INGREDIENTS

- 2 tbsp coconut oil (or your fave alternative)
- 1/8 tsp apple cider vinegar

MAKE IT

1. In a small bowl, mix the coconut oil and apple cider vinegar until well combined. If the coconut oil is solid, warm it gently until it's liquid and smooth. Be sure to ask an adult for help with warming. Let mixture cool.

2. Using clean fingers, apply the mixture to your face in gentle, circular motions. Think of it as a soothing massage for your skin!

3. Rinse your face with warm water and pat dry with a soft towel.

YOU GLOW, GIRL!

Use this tropical treat for your skin a couple of times a week to keep your skin feeling fresh, soft, and oh-so-glowy! Remember that some of these ingredients have acidic qualities, so if it tingles too intensely, go ahead and wash off the mask.

STRAWBABE
LIP SCRUB

Say goodbye to chapped lips and hello to a burst of juicy hydration. Whether you're prepping for your favorite lip gloss or just want a sweet treat for your pout, Strawbabe is here to make your lips feel berry fabulous!

INGREDIENTS

- 1 tbsp honey
- 1 tsp granulated sugar
- 3 strawberries (or your favorite berry)

MAKE IT

1. Pour the honey into a small bowl.
2. Using the back of a spoon, crush the strawberries.
3. Place the crushed strawberries and granulated sugar in the container with the honey and stir into a paste.
4. Use your finger to gently massage the mixture into your lips and leave on for a minute or two. (Safe to eat, sweet, beautifying treat!)
5. Wipe the scrub off with a warm, wet cloth, and pucker your gorgeous glowing pout!

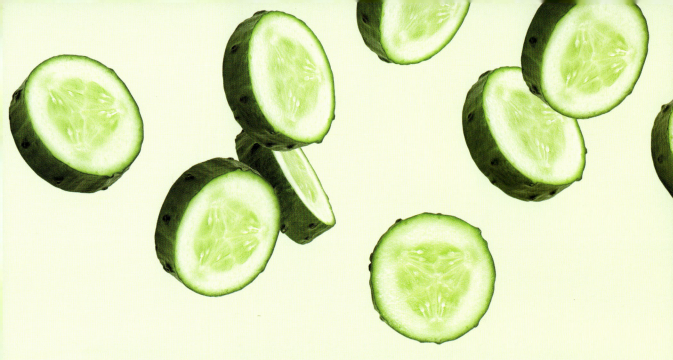

COOLING CUCUMBER
LIP MASK

Give your lips some love with this soothing and hydrating lip mask!

INGREDIENTS

- 1/4 cucumber, sliced
- Shea butter
- Waxelene, Vaseline, or Aquaphor

MAKE IT

1. Place cucumber slices in the fridge to cool.
2. Gently pat your lips dry with a soft cloth.
3. Place a cool cucumber slice on your lips for a few minutes.
4. Apply a thin layer of shea butter to your lips.
5. Top it off with a layer of Waxelene, Vaseline, or Aquaphor to lock in hydration.
6. Let the mask sit overnight for maximum hydration and a perfect pout in the morning!

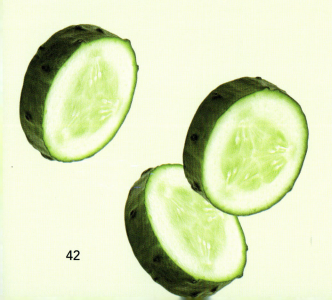

GLOW ON THE GO
LIP BALM

Wanna make your own lip balm? It's totally easy, fun, and perfect for an easy, glossy shine!

INGREDIENTS

- 1 tsp beeswax pellets (or alternative wax)
- 1 tsp coconut oil (or your fave alternatative)
- 1 tsp shea butter

MAKE IT

1. In a small microwave-safe bowl, combine wax, coconut oil, and shea butter. Microwave in 15-second bursts, stirring in between, until it's all melted and smooth. Ask an adult for help with melting.
2. Wait for the mixture to cool. Give it a good stir!
3. Using a steady hand, pour the mixture into an empty lip balm container.
4. Let it cool and harden for about 20 minutes. (Pop it in the fridge if you're impatient like us.)
5. Twist up your homemade balm and enjoy super soft lips!

YOU GLOW, GIRL!

Swipe on and slay. DIY never looked and felt so good!

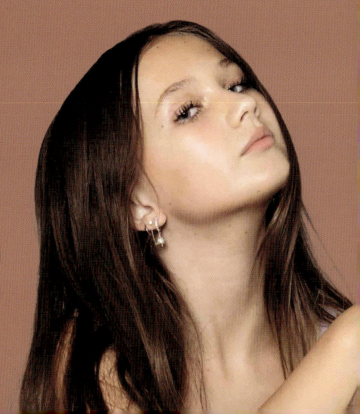

BUSTLING BROWS
EYEBROW SERUM

This luxurious blend of grapeseed, castor, and coconut oils is designed to help your brows look naturally lush and healthy. With each ingredient delivering deep hydration and care, this serum nourishes your brows. Perfect for anyone who loves to highlight their brows, this treatment will leave you feeling good!

INGREDIENTS

- 1 tsp grapeseed oil (or alternative oil)
- 1 tsp castor oil (or alternative oil)
- 1 tsp coconut oil (or alternative oil)

YOU GLOW, GIRL!

You don't have to only use this serum at night — if you prefer, you can wear it during the day. Make sure that you are not allergic or sensitive to any of the oils in this recipe — feel free to use an alternative oil that plays nice with your skin!

MAKE IT

1. In a small, clean container, combine the grapeseed oil, castor oil, and coconut oil. Stir well to create a smooth, silky serum.

2. Using a clean mascara wand or a cotton swab, lightly brush the serum onto your brows, following the natural shape.

3. Leave the serum on overnight to let the oils work their magic. (Tip: Cover your pillowcase with a towel just in case of any extra oil!)

4. In the morning, cleanse your face as usual, gently removing any leftover oil from your brows.

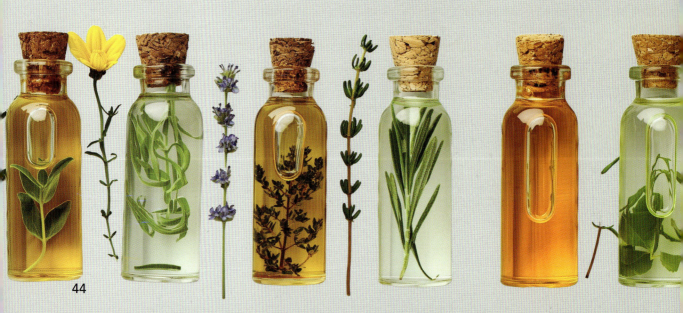

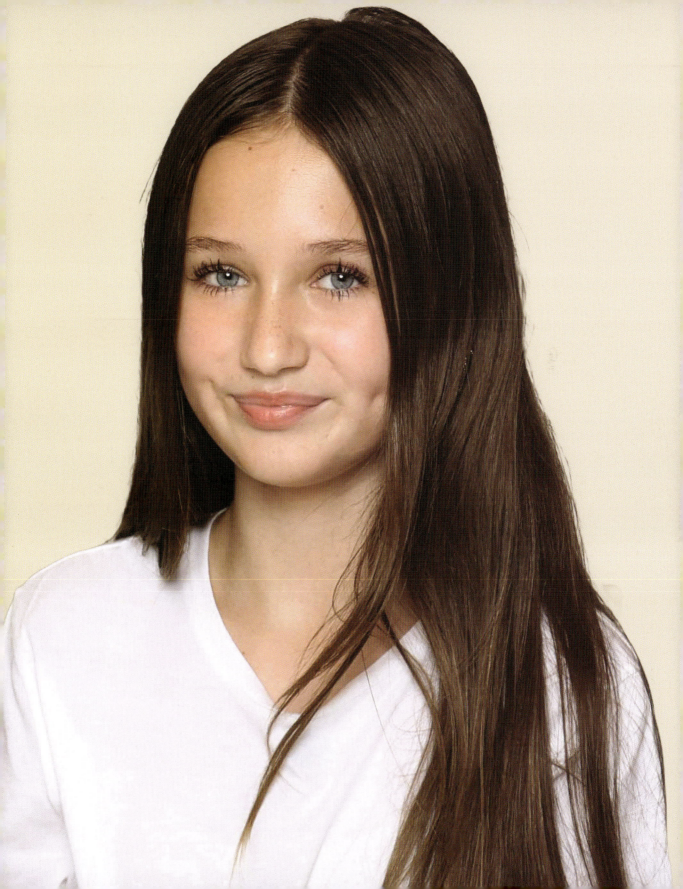

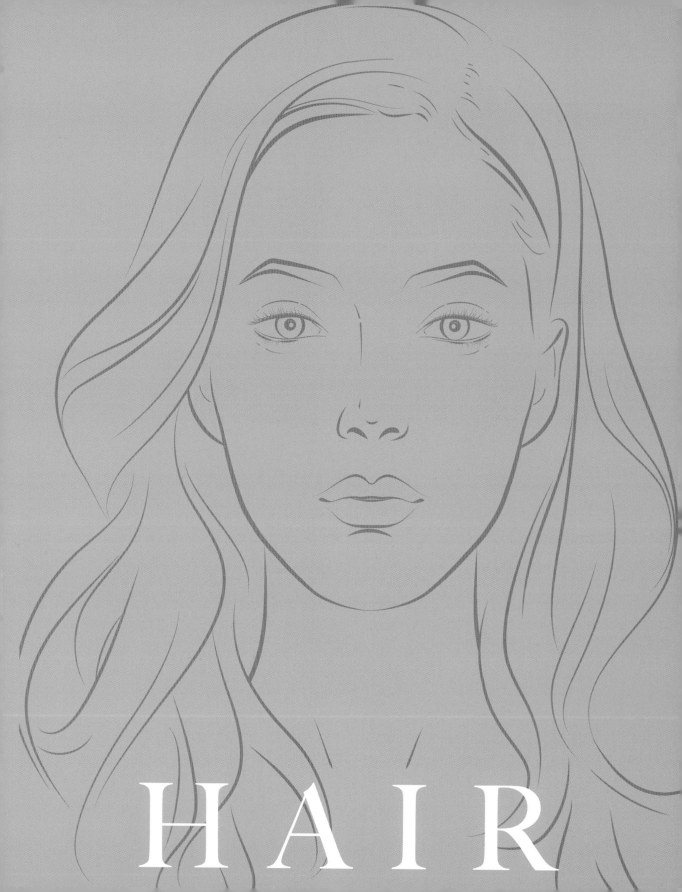

GO, GO AVOCADO
HAIR MASK

Ready to give your locks some love? This DIY avocado hair mask is like a spa day for your hair — hydrating, softening, and totally shiny! Plus, it's super easy to whip up with just a few simple ingredients. Let's get glowing (literally)!

INGREDIENTS

- Half a ripe avocado
- 1 tbsp of your fave conditioner
- 1 tbsp of honey
- Optional: 1/4 banana

MAKE IT

1. Scoop out the avocado and mash it in a bowl until it's nice and creamy. No chunks allowed!
2. Add your conditioner, honey, and banana (if using). Mix it up like you're making guac for your hair — smooth and delicious-looking!
3. Apply generously to your hair, focusing on the ends and any dry areas.
4. Pop on a shower cap (or just chill with a towel around your shoulders), and let this dreamy mask soak in for 20 minutes.
5. Shampoo your hair thoroughly to rinse out the mask. Follow up with your regular conditioner and give your hair a good brush for that final silky touch.

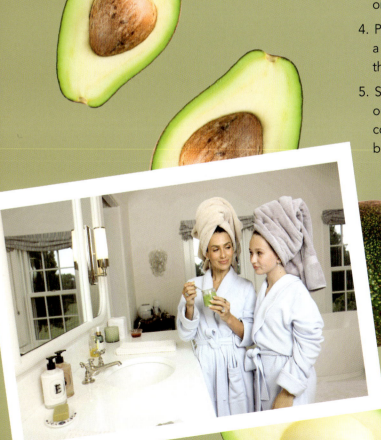

RICE WATER
HAIR MASK

Ready to unlock the ultimate hair secret that's been around forever? Say hello to rice water hair masks! These masks are like a magic potion for shiny, strong hair. Rice water is packed with vitamins and nutrients that can make your hair super soft, super shiny, and just super in general. Let's dive in and give your hair its glow-up moment!

INGREDIENTS

- White rice
- Water
- Blender
- Option 2 requires just the water leftover from cooking rice. (Save it before you drain the rice!)

YOU GLOW, GIRL!

Don't put hot rice water in your hair, wait until it's lukewarm — you don't want to feel like you're cooking it on your head! Use this mask 1–2 times a week for the best results. Too much can make your hair feel stiff. Now go show off your new hair glow to the world — you've earned it!

MAKE IT - OPTION 1

1. Cook your rice with a little extra water so it turns all soft and squishy. Ask an adult for help with this step.
2. Once it's cooked, blend the rice with the extra water until it's smooth and creamy — like a hair smoothie!
3. Shampoo your hair, then apply this mask from roots to tips.
4. Leave it in for 10 minutes, then rinse and condition as usual. Voila — hair magic!

MAKE IT - OPTION 2

1. After cooking your rice, scoop out the starchy water.
2. Once it's cool, pour it all over your hair after shampooing.
3. Leave it on for 10 minutes, then rinse and condition. Run a brush through your now-shiny hair.

SHINY HAIR, I CARE!
REVITALIZING HAIR MASK

With all the TLC your hair needs, this mask is like a spa day in a jar. Whether your locks are feeling dry, frizzy, or just a little meh, this rich formula will breathe new life into every strand, leaving your hair soft, silky, and oh-so-glossy.

INGREDIENTS

- 1/2 cup plain yogurt (or dairy-free alternative)
- 1 tbsp honey
- 1 tbsp olive oil
- 1 tbsp castor oil
- (optional) 1–2 drops rosemary oil
- 1 ripe banana

MAKE IT

1. In a bowl, mash the banana until its free of lumps.
2. Add the plain yogurt to the mashed banana and stir until well blended.
3. Stir in the honey, olive oil, castor oil, and rosemary oil (optional). Mix until everything is smooth and creamy.
4. Section your hair and apply the mask from roots to tips, focusing on ends where your hair seems to be driest.
5. Gently massage the mixture into your scalp.
6. Let it sit — cover your hair with a shower cap or towel and leave the mask on for 20–30 minutes.
7. Rinse out the mask, then shampoo and condition your hair. Run the brush through your hair while conditioning.

SHAKE IT OUT
HAIR DETANGLING SPRAY

Say goodbye to stubborn tangles and hello to silky, manageable locks with this Shake It Out Hair Detangling Spray! Perfect for all hair types, this easy DIY recipe combines the gentle power of your favorite conditioner with optional essential oils to soften strands and make brushing a breeze. It's lightweight, smells amazing, and is free from harsh chemicals — because your hair deserves nothing but the best!

INGREDIENTS

- 2 tbsp conditioner
- 1 cup warm water
- (optional) 1–2 drops essential oil

MAKE IT

1. In a clean mixing bowl, whisk together the conditioner and warm water until fully blended. The warm water helps the conditioner dissolve more easily.
2. Stir in the essential oil of your choice (if oils are your thing). Lavender is great for relaxation, rosemary can promote hair growth, and tea tree oil helps maintain a healthy scalp.
3. Pour the mixture into a clean spray bottle using a funnel to avoid spills.
4. Cap the bottle tightly and shake well to ensure the ingredients are evenly mixed.
5. Spray a couple spritzes onto damp or dry hair, focusing on the ends and any tangles. Gently comb through with a wide-tooth comb or your fingers.

YOU GLOW, GIRL!

Always shake the bottle before use to remix the ingredients. For an extra boost, store the spray in the fridge for a refreshing, soothing detangling experience. With every spritz, your hair will feel softer, shinier, and more manageable. Time to shake it out and let your hair shine!

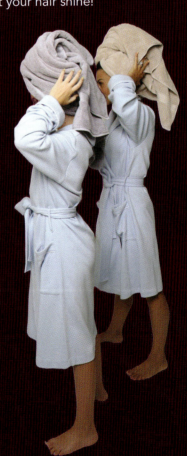

SCRUB AWAY THE BLUES
SCALP SCRUB

Your scalp deserves just as much love as the rest of your skin! This Scrub Away the Stress Scalp Scrub is the perfect way to refresh your roots, remove buildup, and stimulate healthy hair growth. With exfoliating sugar, nourishing oil, invigorating essential oils, and balancing apple cider vinegar, this scrub not only soothes your scalp but also leaves your hair feeling fresh and rejuvenated.

INGREDIENTS

- 1/4 cup sugar
- 2 tbsp oil of your choice
- (optional) 1–2 drops essential oil
- 1/8 tsp apple cider vinegar

MAKE IT

1. In a small bowl, combine the sugar and oil. Stir until the sugar is evenly coated.
2. Mix in the essential oil (optional) and apple cider vinegar, stirring until fully incorporated. The texture should be grainy but moist enough to spread.
3. Apply to a damp scalp, parting your hair in sections. Gently massage the scrub into your scalp with your fingertips for 2–3 minutes.
4. Rinse thoroughly with warm water and follow with your regular shampoo and conditioner.
5. Run the brush through your hair while conditioning.

YOU GLOW, GIRL!

Use once a week for best results. For extra relaxation, massage the scrub into your scalp while taking deep breaths to enjoy the soothing scent of the essential oils. Avoid applying too much pressure to prevent irritation — gentle circular motions work best.

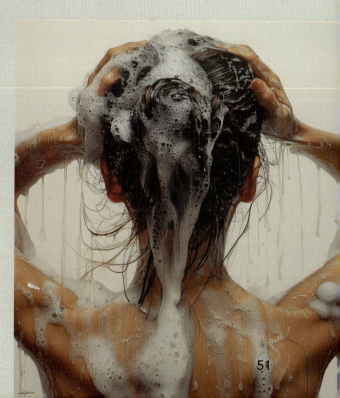

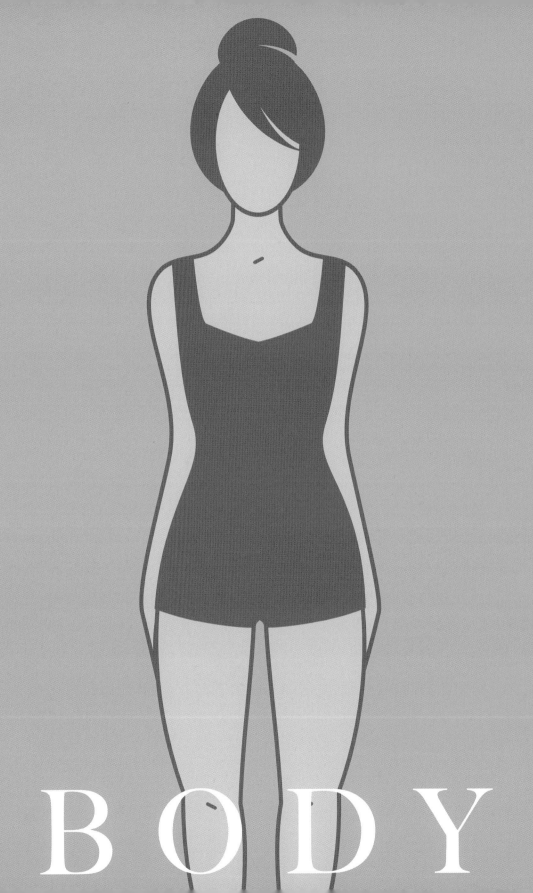

SILKY SMOOTH
BODY SCRUB

With gentle sugar crystals for exfoliation, and a dash of your favorite body wash for lather, this scrub feels like pure bliss in a jar. Perfect for a little self-care moment, this custom scrub will leave your skin feeling polished, refreshed, and oh-so-silky.

INGREDIENTS

- 1/2 cup sugar
- 1/4 cup your favorite body wash

MAKE IT

1. In a small bowl, combine the sugar and body wash. Stir until it forms a thick, scrubby consistency.

2. In the shower, scoop a small amount of scrub into your hand and gently massage onto damp skin in circular motions, focusing on areas that need extra love, like elbows, knees, and heels. DO NOT use this scrub on your face.

3. Rinse off with warm water to reveal soft, smooth skin.

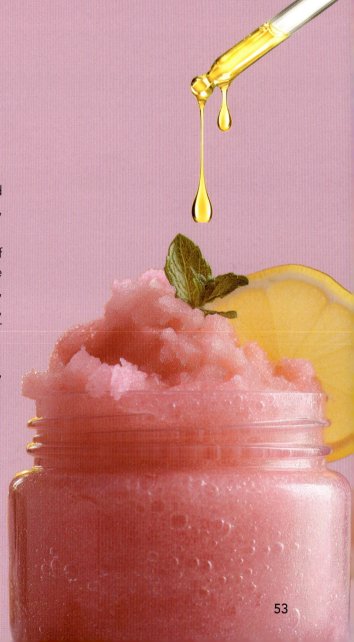

DREAMY FEET
FOOT MASK

Get ready for the ultimate pamper session for your tired toes! With a hydrating base of Vaseline (or Waxelene/Aquaphor), a splash of olive oil, and a hint of soothing essential oils, this foot mask is like a cozy blanket for your feet. Perfect for those nights when your feet need extra TLC, this mask will leave them feeling softer, smoother, and ready to step into a new day!

INGREDIENTS

- 1 tbsp Vaseline, Waxelene, or Aquaphor
- 1/2 tsp olive oil
- (optional) 1 drop of essential oil
- cotton socks

MAKE IT

1. In a small bowl, blend the Vaseline (or your preferred base), olive oil, and essential oil until smooth and creamy.
2. Before bed, slather the mixture onto clean, dry feet, giving extra attention to heels and rough areas. Don't stand up; your feet are slippery!
3. Slip on a pair of soft cotton socks to lock in the moisture while you sleep and let the mask work its magic overnight.
4. In the morning, remove your socks and rinse your feet with warm water. Remember your feet might still be slippery, so be careful!

YOU GLOW, GIRL!

Enjoy this luxurious mask once a week, and get ready to step out with softer, happier feet!

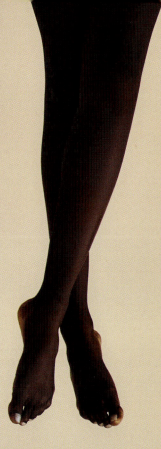
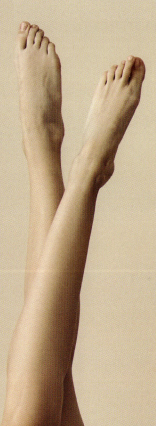

NOURISHED NAILS
NAIL & CUTICLE OIL

This is a quick and easy way to keep your nails and cuticles soft, healthy, and ready to shine! This blend of coconut oil and sunflower oil delivers deep hydration and natural nutrients to strengthen your nails and condition your cuticles. Perfect for a little self-care moment, this oil is lightweight, nourishing, and easy to apply.

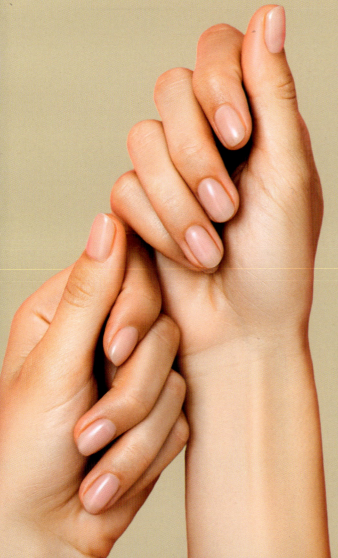

INGREDIENTS

- 1 tsp coconut oil (or your favorite alternative oil)
- 1 tsp sunflower oil

MAKE IT

1. In a small, clean container, mix together the coconut oil and sunflower oil until well blended. You can adjust the quantities if you'd like to make a larger batch!

2. Apply a small amount of oil to each nail and massage gently into the cuticles. Let it absorb fully for soft, happy cuticles and nails!

3. Use daily or as needed, especially after washing your hands, to keep your nails and cuticles hydrated and healthy.

YOU GLOW, GIRL!

Your nails will feel stronger, and your cuticles will stay nourished and smooth — perfect for maintaining salon-fresh hands!

SWEET AS HONEY
MILK BATH

Want to soak like royalty? This Honey Milk Bath is a luxurious treat that'll leave your skin super soft and oh-so-glowy! Cleopatra loved milk baths, and now you can too — because every queen deserves a little pampering! And don't worry — if you're dairy-free, just use your favorite milk alternative!

INGREDIENTS

- 1 cup milk (or your favorite milk alternative!)
- 1/4 cup honey

YOU GLOW, GIRL!

Soak up the goodness, and let your skin feel as sweet as honey!

MAKE IT

1. Warm the milk slightly (just so it blends better with the honey — no need to boil!). Ask an adult for help with warming.
2. Stir in the honey until it's all mixed and dreamy.
3. Pour into your warm bath and swirl the water to mix.
4. Slide in, relax, and let your skin soak up all the softness!

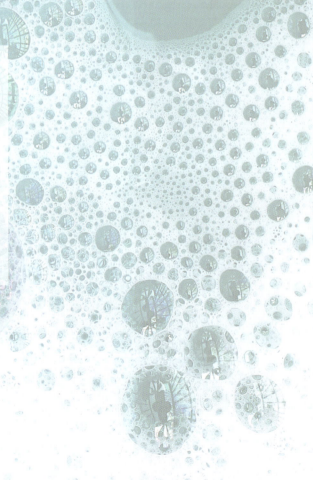

TROPICAL GLOW
SUGAR SCRUB

Hey, sunshine! Ready to get silky smooth skin that feels like you just stepped off a tropical beach? This Coconut Sugar Scrub is your new BFF for soft, glowing skin! It gently scrubs away dry skin while keeping you moisturized and glowing — plus, it smells AH-MAZING! Bonus? It's super easy to make! Let's get glowing!

INGREDIENTS

- 1/2 cup coconut oil (or any other skin-friendly oil if needed!)
- 1/2 cup sugar

MAKE IT

1. Soften the coconut oil by rubbing it between your hands. Once it's soft, transfer into a small bowl.
2. Mix in the sugar until it looks like a magical, sandy scrub!
3. Gently massage onto damp skin in circles — focus on rough spots like elbows, knees, and heels!
4. Rinse off and pat dry for super soft, happy skin!

YOU GLOW, GIRL!

Add a spoonful of cocoa powder for a deliciously chocolate-scented body treat! Now go glow like the beach goddess you are!

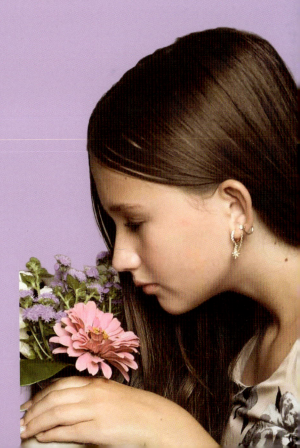

BANISH THOSE BLUES
HYDRATING BODY OIL

Life can sometimes feel a little heavy, but your skincare doesn't have to! This Banish Those Blues Hydrating Body Oil is cozy and nurturing — light and infused with mood-boosting ingredients to hydrate your skin and lift your spirits. Whether you're facing a tough day or simply need a pick-me-up, this luxurious oil is here to brighten your mood and leave your skin glowing.

INGREDIENTS

- 4 tsp sunflower oil
- 2 tsp olive oil
- 2 tsp coconut oil (or alternative oil)
- (optional) 1 drop lavendar essential oil

MAKE IT

1. Using a funnel, pour oils into the glass bottle. Add essential oil. Shake before each use.

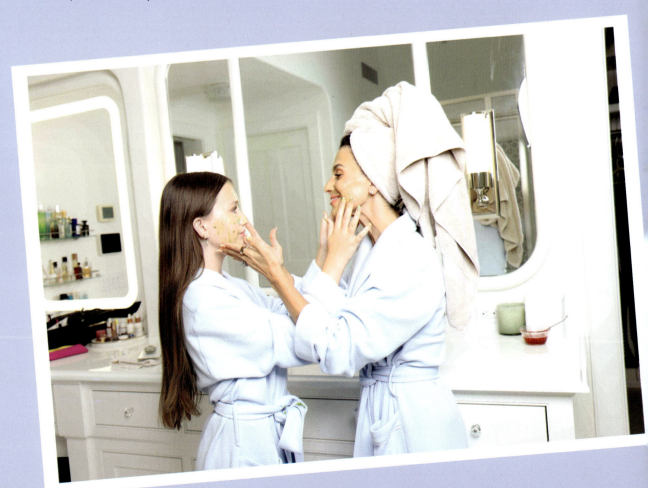

SASSY SUDS
SHOWER GEL

Turn your shower into a sassy spa experience with this Sassy Suds Shower Gel! Packed with gentle, nourishing ingredients, this DIY recipe leaves your skin feeling soft, smooth, and oh-so-clean. The combination of moisturizing honey, soothing oils, and a hint of salt for balance ensures your skin stays hydrated while enjoying a rich, bubbly lather.

INGREDIENTS

- 3/4 cup your fave body wash
- 1–2 tsp oil of choice or liquid aloe vera
- 2 tbsp honey

MAKE IT

1. Add the body wash, oil or aloe vera, and honey to the bowl. Stir gently to combine, avoiding excessive foaming.
2. Continue mixing until all ingredients are well incorporated, and the texture is smooth.
3. Pour the mixture into a clean pump or squeeze bottle using a funnel.
4. In the shower, pump a small amount onto a loofah, sponge, or directly onto your hands. Lather up, rinse off, and revel in your skin's softness!

YOU GLOW, GIRL!

Store your shower gel in a cool, dry place and shake gently before each use to keep the ingredients well mixed. Get ready to sass up your shower routine and step out feeling fabulous, refreshed, and ready to conquer the day!

LUXURIATE
LOTION

Pamper your skin with this Luxurious Lotion, the ultimate treat for dry or sensitive skin! Made with a heavenly combo of coconut oil and shea butter, this lotion delivers deep hydration and a protective barrier against dryness. Also perfect for on-the-go moisture or as a thoughtful handmade gift!

INGREDIENTS

- 4 oz coconut oil (or alternative oil)
- 4 oz shea butter
- (optional) 1–5 drops essential oils
- 1 tsp vitamin E oil

YOU GLOW, GIRL!

With this luscious lotion, your skin will feel pampered, protected, and irresistibly soft — every day!

MAKE IT

1. Combine the coconut oil, shea butter, and vitamin E oil in a heat-safe microwave bowl. Heat gently over low heat, stirring occasionally, until fully melted and blended. Ask an adult for help with this step.
2. Remove from heat and let the mixture cool (but not solidify). Stir in any optional essential oils or vitamin E oil.
3. Carefully pour the mixture into a small container of your choice. Ask an adult to help you with this step also.
4. Let the mixture cool for 1–2 hours.
5. Gently rub lotion over your skin for luxurious, long-lasting moisture.

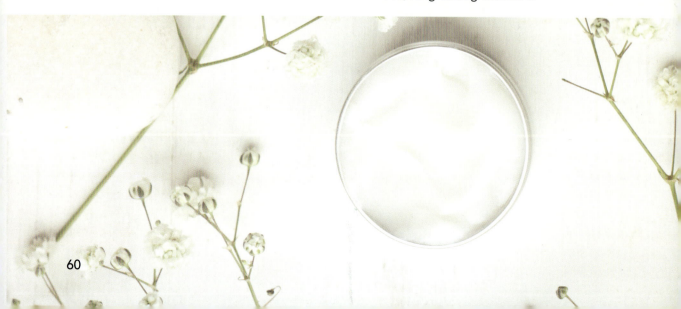

DERMATOLOGIST APPROVED

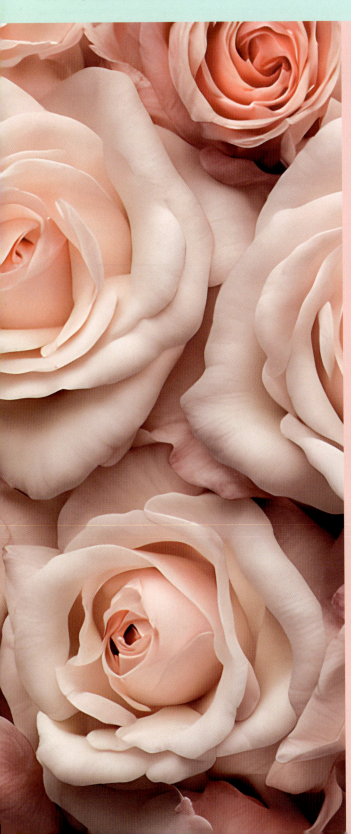

Hey there, future skin care experts! If you're like most teens, your skin is going through a lot right now. Those pesky breakouts, the oily shine, and the occasional sensitivity – it can all be a bit frustrating. But don't worry, because I've got some good news: using the right skincare products can make a huge difference.

Here's why teen-specific skincare is so important:

Your skin is different: Teen skin is still developing, and it's much more sensitive than adult skin. Harsh ingredients found in adult products can irritate your skin, leading to dryness, redness, and even more breakouts.

Hormones are the culprit: Those crazy hormones are responsible for the increased oil production that clogs your pores and causes acne. Teen-focused skincare often contains ingredients like salicylic acid or tea tree oil, which help unclog pores without over-drying your skin.

Sun protection is key: Sun damage at a young age can have serious long-term consequences, like premature aging and skin cancer. Teen-specific skincare lines prioritize broad-spectrum sun protection with high SPF, helping you stay safe in the sun and prevent future damage.

Build good habits early: Starting a good skincare routine in your teens can set you up for a lifetime of healthy skin. By addressing your concerns now and learning how to care for your skin properly, you'll develop habits that will benefit you for years to come.

So, what are you waiting for? It's time to take control of your skin and start using products that are specifically designed for your needs. Your skin will thank you later!

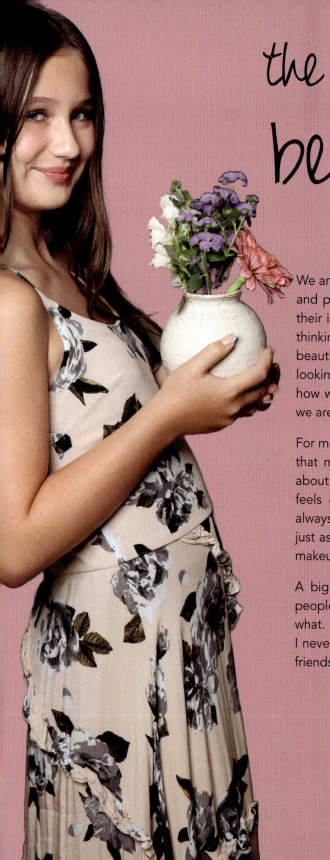

the secret is... being YOU!

We are surrounded by images of other people's lives, and pressured to constantly comparing ourselves to their idea of "pretty." It's easy to fall into the trap of thinking you need to look like someone else to feel beautiful. But here's the truth: beauty isn't about looking a certain way. Living a beautiful life is about how we feel inside and out. Makeup or no makeup, we are amazing just the way we are.

For me, I always try to express who I am. I've learned that makeup isn't about changing who I am — it's about celebrating and sharing myself in a way that feels good to me. It's my self-expression, and it's always changing. And honestly? I love that I can feel just as much like myself with a bare face as I do with makeup on.

A big part of that confidence comes from having people in my life who always support me, no matter what. From tomboy to experimenting with makeup, I never feel like I am being judged by my family and friends for expressing myself.

I had a tomboy phase where I hated wearing dresses. I also remember using lipstick to draw on my face, and using face paint as if it were makeup.

I have so much fun experimenting, with no specific goal in mind other than to do what makes me feel good. It's not about trying to fit in or impress anyone — I am just figuring out what makes me happy. And that's the best advice I can give: try new things and see what feels right for you.

The coolest part about experimenting is that it's our own journey. We don't have to look or act like anyone else. Every time we try something new, whether it's clothes or makeup, we're just discovering another way to be ourselves. And remember, we are all on our own path. Just because someone else looks or acts differently doesn't make them — or you or me — any less amazing!

As we're growing up, we won't always know exactly who we are or who we want to become. It's a process of figuring ourselves out, and learning to embrace ourselves along the way.

Remember, there is no "perfect" way to do anything; as long as it works for you, you're doing it right!

LET'S TALK ABOUT LEARNING TO PAPMER YOURSELF

Hilaria

Carmen and her siblings are growing up in a household where curiosity is encouraged, so questions have turned into experiments, and experiments turn into phases. Self-expression is revered and we want them to have reasonable freedom to try new things. It is important that they feel happy in their skin as they grow, and that they find ways to express how they feel on the outside with every change.

Carmen

When I first started playing with makeup, I was a toddler and in love with the idea of having bright colors on my face. I used blue lipstick to draw on my face, or I'd choose to have bright red lips, and not know how to keep the color just on my lips . . . which makes me cringe when I think back on it. I guess it was cute, and I think it's cute when my younger siblings do this too. Even if I regret some of those choices now, I'm glad that I was given space for my expression!

Makeup and self-care have always been one of the ways that I like to express my creativity and show my personality. While I have fun with makeup and skincare, I know it's a tool for self-expression that I like and feels right for me, and it's not right for everyone. Just do what feels right for you. No one should shame you for your choices with your life and your body. And you should never feel pressured to do something or not do something, be a certain way or not be a certain way.

I feel more myself when I take "me time," like my mom, and I love it so much that I hope everyone can take the time to feel this way by having fun with pampering yourself. It's about feeling good and feeling you!

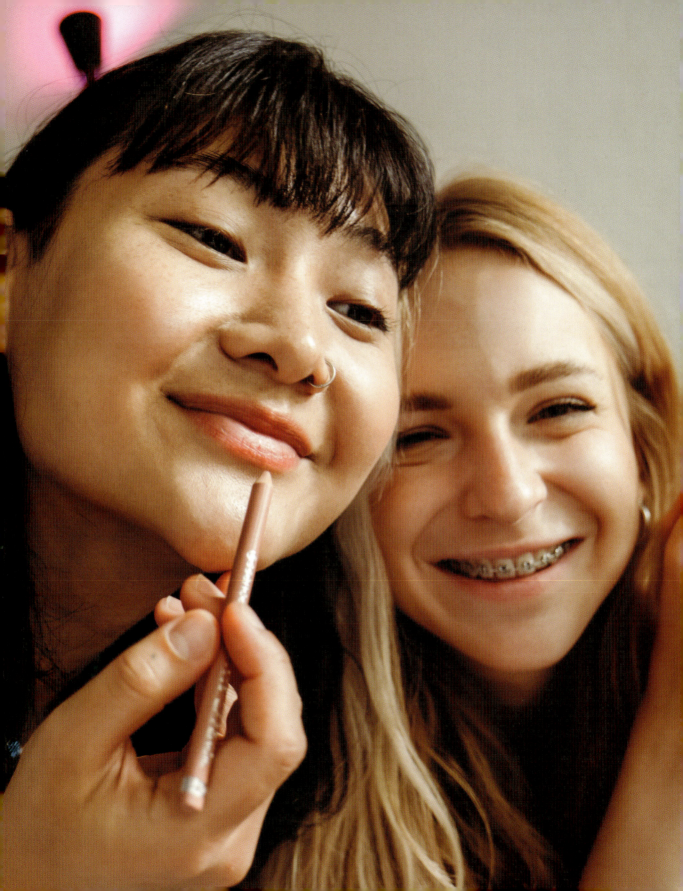

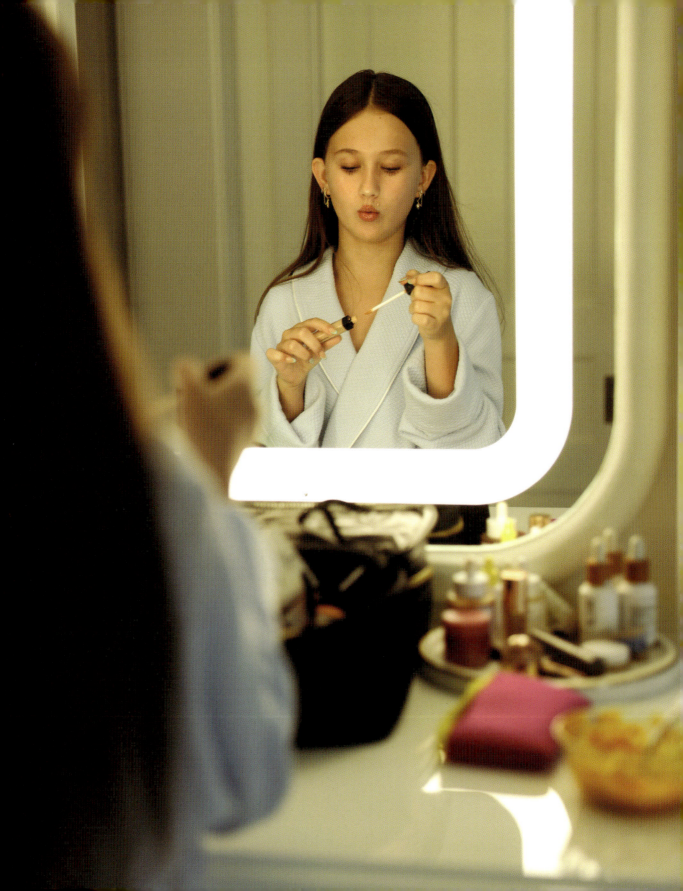

SKINCARE IS SELF CARE

I started really getting into skincare two years ago, when I was nine, even though I had always played with makeup to some extent. Now, I've got a routine that makes my skin feel healthy and glowing, and it's one of my favorite ways to practice self-care.

My mom tells me that as I grow up and my skin changes, my routine and the products I use will change too. I have a really good skincare routine that works well for my skin, and I am always experimenting and creating more. It's lots of trial and error and lots of fun. It's about playing and having fun and noticing what feels good. Everyone's skin is different, and I am learning that everyone's skin may be different year by year as well.

You may not be asking for my advice, but if you are . . . My advice for starting a skincare routine is to first start small. Don't start with five products and expect to know what works and what doesn't. I've done this and I don't recommend it!

I learned to try new things, little by little and always focus on the ingredients. Even if things are natural too, not everyone can use the same products. You have to be your own skin expert, and there are safe ways to customize each recipe. Like my little sister, Marilu, she can't use anything with almonds. We all have to be careful and talk to our parents and doctors. Once we know what ingredients work for our skin, sunscreen, masks, and moisturizers are such great ways to pamper ourselves and nourish and protect our skin!

Skincare and makeup are so popular with kids my age. Since I was young, my mom has always been conscious of the ingredients of things that we use. Food, products, medicines — everything!

It isn't like we're a 100% natural household. I use homemade hair masks, but I also use storebought shampoo to wash my hair. I've been taught the importance of balancing both things — and making sure we know of anything that might be harmful in each thing.

I'll admit that I've had some bad experiences with both homemade products and with storebought products, so I've learned the hard way (like when I turned my dad orange — aren't you glad he was my test subject?). It's important to pay attention to ingredients and what's safe — and not staining.

While I love storebought products too, I do love making my own natural stuff at home. It's usually just better for your skin, and you don't have to stress about mystery chemicals.

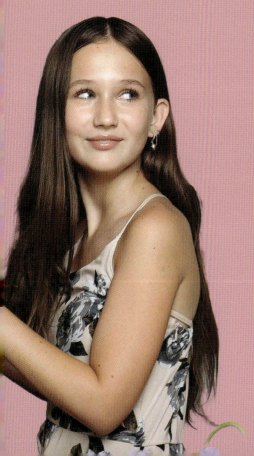

For people who are new to skincare and want to buy products instead of making them yourself, I would highly suggest you do your research on everything before trying it out on your skin. My rule is not to trust anything without checking it out first. And I don't mean just reading the labels; I mean looking at what other people have said about the product!

Reviews are important, because they're from real people like me and you who are using the products. You can look for people with your same skin or hair type to get the best idea of how it will affect you. You have to be thorough unless you want to learn the hard way.

I use an app called Yuka, where you can scan a product's barcode to see its rating and reviews. I've even added info to the app to help others out because it's hard to tell what's good or bad just by looking at the packaging, and honestly,

Carmen

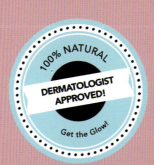

KNOW WHAT'S IN YOUR PRODUCTS

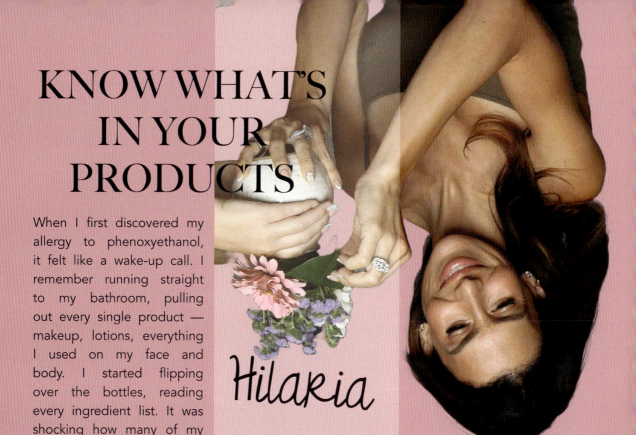

When I first discovered my allergy to phenoxyethanol, it felt like a wake-up call. I remember running straight to my bathroom, pulling out every single product — makeup, lotions, everything I used on my face and body. I started flipping over the bottles, reading every ingredient list. It was shocking how many of my trusted products contained something I was allergic to, something I didn't even know to look for before. That day, I threw out so much, but it was also the start of a new habit: I now check the label on everything before I buy or use it.

This habit has become a huge part of how I approach skin and hair care, and it's something I've started teaching Carmen, too. She loves using her little products — face masks, lip balms, lotions, perfume — and I want her to understand how important it is to know what's in them. Just because something is marketed a certain way doesn't mean it's entirely truthful. Words like "natural," "clean," or "gentle" can be so misleading. Brands know how to sell, and sometimes they're not giving you the full picture.

I've explained to Carmen that what you put on your skin doesn't just stay on the surface. Your skin absorbs it, and it goes into your body. It's so important to be mindful of this, especially when it comes to products we use every day. By teaching her to read labels now, I hope I'm giving her the tools to make informed choices as she grows. It's about being vigilant, not fearful, and understanding what works for your unique body.

Taking the time to know what's in the products you use isn't just an act of self-care — it's an act of self-respect. It's about creating a routine that prioritizes your health and wellbeing, and for me, it's also about setting an example for my children. What we put on our skin matters, and when we pay attention to the details, we're making an investment in ourselves and in the people we love.

NATURAL INGREDIENTS

There's something so satisfying about mixing up a treatment that's uniquely yours. To help you get started, here's a list of other natural ingredients from across the globe that you can explore. Let your creativity shine and see what works best for your skin.

In every part of the world, natural ingredients have been treasured for generations to enhance beauty and care for the skin. Shea butter from West Africa is deeply nourishing. In the Amazon rainforest, antioxidant-packed cacao is a go-to. The Middle East embraces argan oil for its hydrating and anti-aging properties. Jojoba oil, sourced from arid regions, provides balancing hydration. Coconut oil, a staple in Pacific cultures, is a versatile solution for skin and hair care. These timeless ingredients not only highlight nature's power in beauty but also remind us of the deep connections shared through global skincare rituals. The possibilities are endless, so have fun and explore what speaks to you!

Rice Water: Rich in vitamins and antioxidants, rice water brightens skin, improves elasticity, softens, and reduces inflammation for a radiant complexion.

Green Tea: Packed with catechins, this antioxidant-rich tea reduces redness, combats acne, fights free radicals, and soothes skin inflammation effectively.

Matcha (Powdered Green Tea): High in antioxidants, matcha rejuvenates skin, fights acne, reduces redness, and detoxifies for a brighter, clearer complexion.

Ginseng: Boosts circulation, enhances elasticity, and brightens dull skin while rejuvenating and nourishing for a youthful appearance.

Seaweed: Rich in minerals and nutrients, seaweed detoxifies, hydrates, and rejuvenates skin while improving overall texture and tone.

Yuzu (Japanese Citrus): Packed with vitamin C, yuzu brightens skin, boosts collagen, and evens tone for a youthful, radiant appearance.

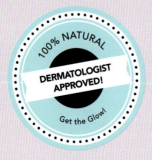

AROUND THE GLOBE

Mung Beans: Mung beans gently exfoliate, reduce acne, and soothe irritation, promoting clear, smooth, and healthy-looking skin.

Shea Butter: Rich in vitamins A and E, shea butter deeply hydrates, reduces inflammation, and aids healing for soft, nourished skin.

Black Soap (Ose Dudu): This natural cleanser exfoliates, clears acne, fades dark spots, and cleanses deeply without harsh chemicals.

Baobab Oil: Rich in omega fatty acids and antioxidants, baobab oil hydrates deeply, reduces dryness, and improves skin elasticity.

Marula Oil: Lightweight and fast-absorbing, marula oil hydrates, protects against environmental damage, and softens skin.

Argan Oil: Rich in vitamin E and fatty acids, argan oil nourishes, reduces scars, and promotes elasticity for smooth, radiant skin.

Rooibos (Red Bush Tea): Loaded with antioxidants, rooibos fights free radicals, reduces inflammation, and soothes skin while improving its overall health.

Rhassoul Clay: Mineral-rich clay detoxifies skin, tightens pores, and absorbs excess oil while gently cleansing and balancing.

Kalahari Melon Seed Oil: Lightweight and non-comedogenic, this oil hydrates, regulates sebum production, and is perfect for acne-prone skin.

Olive Oil: Full of antioxidants, vitamins, and fatty acids, olive oil nourishes, hydrates, and protects skin while restoring moisture.

Rose Water: Soothing and hydrating, rose water balances pH levels, reduces redness, and refreshes with a light, calming scent.

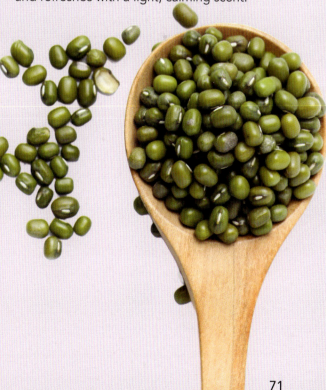

NATURAL INGREDIENTS

Chamomile: Calms irritation and reduces redness with anti-inflammatory properties, promoting soft, soothed, and radiant skin.

Sea Salt: Mineral-rich sea salt detoxifies skin, balances oil production, and gently exfoliates for a refreshed, healthy glow.

Lavender: Anti-inflammatory and calming, lavender soothes sensitive skin, reduces redness, and promotes a balanced, clear complexion.

Cucumber: Hydrating and refreshing, cucumber reduces puffiness, brightens skin, and soothes irritation for a fresh, revitalized look.

Apple Cider Vinegar: With natural astringent properties, apple cider vinegar tones skin, balances pH, and reduces breakouts effectively.

Açai Berries: Loaded with vitamins A, C, and E, açai berries protect skin from environmental damage and boost radiance with antioxidants.

Camu Camu: This vitamin C powerhouse promotes collagen production, brightens skin tone, and reduces hyperpigmentation for glowing skin.

Papaya: Papain enzymes in papaya gently exfoliate dead cells, improve texture, and brighten for smooth, radiant skin.

Avocado: Packed with healthy fats, vitamins, and antioxidants, avocado deeply moisturizes and rejuvenates dry, tired skin.

Yerba Mate: Rich in caffeine and antioxidants, yerba mate firms skin, reduces puffiness, and refreshes for a youthful appearance.

Clay: Mineral-rich clays detoxify, absorb excess oil, and purify for balanced, clear skin with reduced pore appearance.

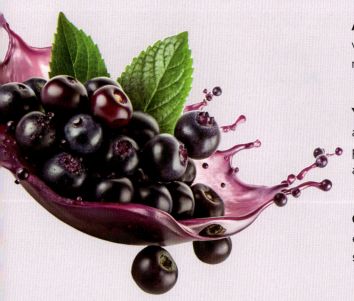

AROUND THE GLOBE

Rosehip Oil: Rich in vitamin A and fatty acids, rosehip oil reduces scars, fine lines, and discoloration for even, smooth skin.

Coffee Grounds: Caffeine improves circulation and reduces puffiness while exfoliating to leave skin smooth and invigorated.

Cacao: Loaded with flavonoids, cacao hydrates, fights free radicals, and nourishes skin, leaving it soft and radiant.

Neem: Antibacterial, antifungal, and anti-inflammatory properties make neem ideal for treating acne, irritation, and maintaining clear skin.

Cedarwood: Anti-inflammatory and antiseptic cedarwood reduces irritation, treats acne, and supports healing for calm, balanced skin.

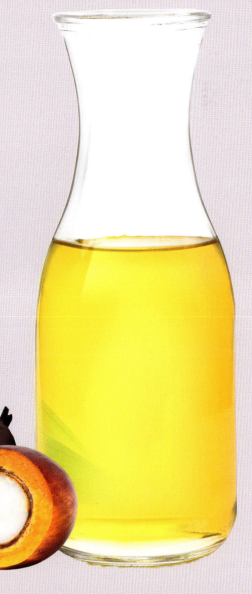

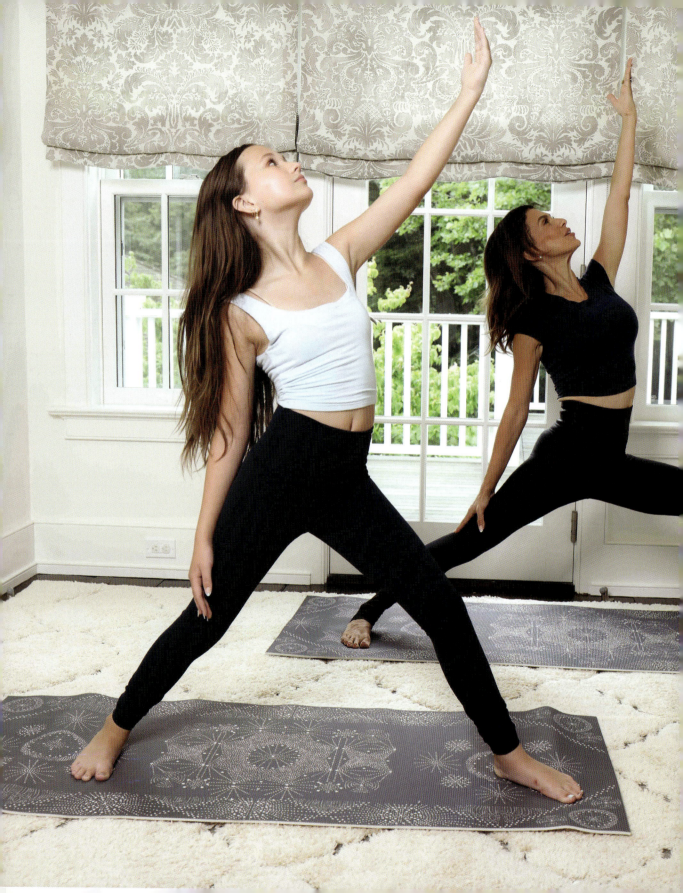

GLOWING UP

LET'S SKIP TO THE GOOD PART

Like so many parents, I wish I could bubblewrap my kids and have them just enjoy being innocent children. Obviously, this is impossible, and part of growing up is learning to exist and thrive in a world that is not always easy and kind. There is so much good, but the bad can be very painful. Raising children in the age of social media is particularly scary and a whole new challenge for us being parents right now. Whether our child has social media or not, they are undoubtably exposed to some of it or its influence on our culture and their peers. Filters, lighting, "perfect" curation, merchandizing, unattainable and weird made up "beauty" standards. It's hard not to compare their real life to someone's curated, online one.

As girls and women, we unfortunately have the capacity to be pros at the comparison game, which isn't great for the whole "feeling good about yourself" thing we are trying to instill in our kids. Sometimes as grown women, we can still be so immature and plain old toxic. We can also be insecure and intimidated by others, regardless of the other person's intention. It's no wonder, since society has raised us with so much judgment and fear.

We are encouraged to covet being the the "prettiest," "smartest," "funniest," and most "liked." It's exhausting. Not only is this impossible because all of the "ests" are made up, but it also means that if someone is "the fairest of them all," everyone else, by default, has to be less than her. It's not good for any of us.

Trying to fit into impossible and made-up boxes of "beauty" and "behavior" is miserable and inevitably impossible. We can pretend, but it means we cannot show our real selves, and we should never have to mask, nor expect our children to. We all know how painful this is and can be. That "good girl" mentality is based off of fear, and I for one, want to raise a fearless daughter. None of this, "Be smart, but don't be a know-it-all. Be strong, but not so strong you scare people. Be yourself, but make sure you're relatable." Can't we just live?

What if we just cut it out and skip to the good part? An embrace of, "my humanity sees and honors your humanity and I want you to be free and happy. I want me to be free and happy." We all want our daughters to be free and happy.

The good news? We are raising our daughters in a time when we can talk about these things more openly. This conversation is one of the reasons I am most excited for this book. The more we put this free and happy out there, the more it hopefully spreads.

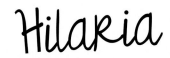

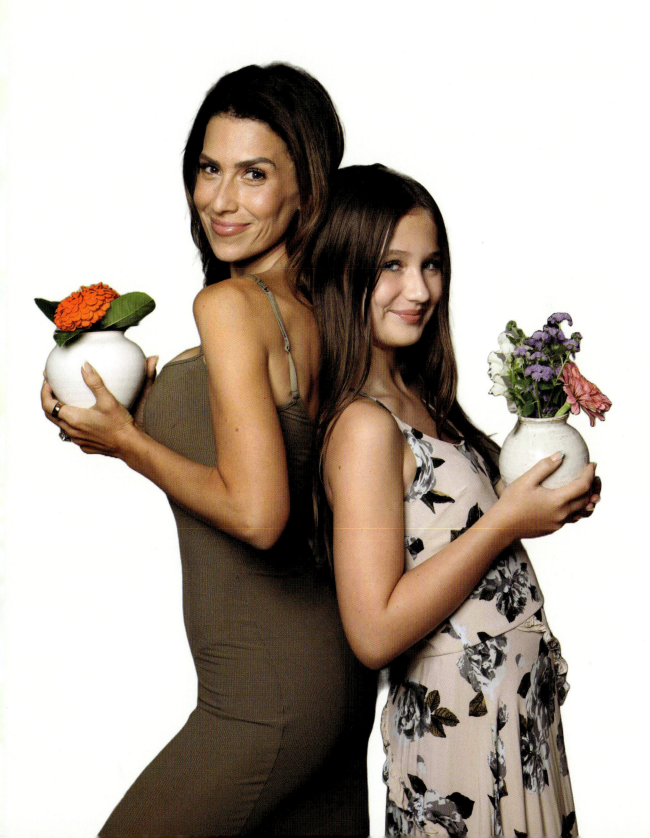

My mom is my best friend. I don't say that just to say it. I have seen her go through a lot and she has seen me go through a lot. No matter how hard our days are, or what we are dealing with, we are such a good team. We always say that in our house: somos un buen equipo. We are a good team. Most of the time we are having fun, but we are not always going to agree and get along. When this happens, we know we can always work it out, telling each other that even with the best of intentions, we will not get it right all the time.

I know she is always there for me. She wants me to be happy and this is why I feel safe telling her anything. She never judges me, She just reminds me of who I am and that I will find my way. I am never alone and she is always there to be my friend and my mom. If I say anything mean about myself, she disagrees and reassures me that this is normal for anyone, but it doesn't make it okay to be mean to yourself. She makes me feel better knowing that we all have insecurities, and we can always feel better when we talk about them and learn what they really are about. I have learned from her that sometimes our fears lie to us. She calls these "tricky" feelings, meaning they are feelings that trick us to feeling badly, when there is no reason to. It is hard sometimes to separate the tricky ones and the real ones. My mom is a yoga teacher, so she will say something that annoys me like: it's a process!

Then she will often make the same cringey joke: "I made you. Be nice to the things I made."

As much as I roll my eyes at her sometimes, my mom and I are always in each other's corner. My mom is my best friend.

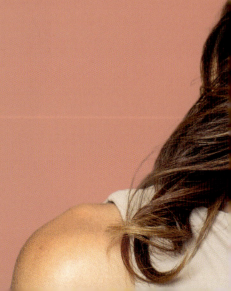

I started playing with makeup and skincare because of dress up. Now it's become another thing that my mom and I bond over. We have a lot of things that we do together, and this is just another thing that we share. It's been fun to work with her to pick out the best products for me and for her. I have taught her a lot and I love that she actually listens to me and makes changes. Sometimes she lets me do a facial on her and she is always asking for advice on how to apply makeup like I do.

She teaches me by pointing out which products have harsh chemicals that we need to avoid, and she has made sure that I know how to find products that have natural ingredients that are good for my skin.

She always encourages me to explore by supporting my artistic expressions, even if that meant getting very messy . . . or the house getting very messy.

Carmen

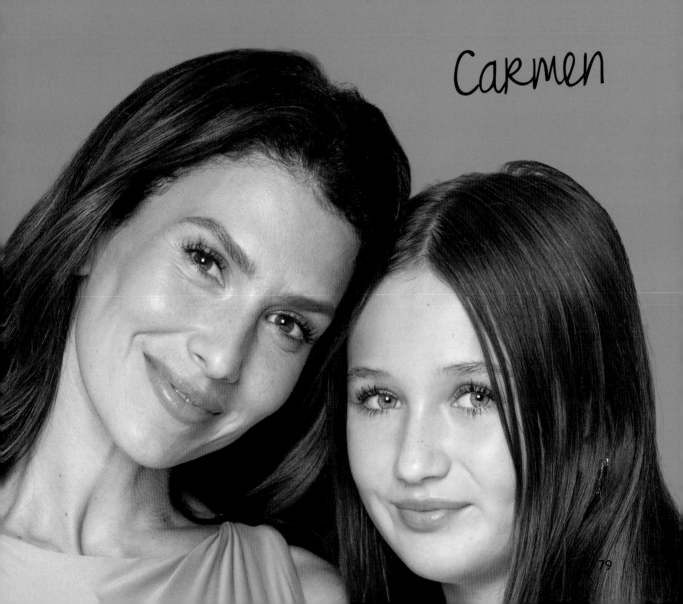

One of my favorite things about having had so many children is I really got to see, firsthand, how they each come out with their own unique soul and are such little individuals. Children truly are such remarkable little beings. If you take a moment to step back and just watch, you can see their personalities shine through in the most amazing ways. They're all so full of spirit, and it's such a privilege to witness.

Carmen, for example, has always been outgoing and silly — she's her father's daughter in so many ways. She has this clownish side that loves to make people laugh, and she's really good at it, too. Like all kids, she loves to feel seen, heard, and appreciated. She is just as good at making others feel that way. We speak a lot about empathy and humanity, in our family. I hope that my children always carry this with them.

There's a poem by Kahlil Gibran, "On Children," that has always resonated with me. It's such a beautiful reminder that our children are here to be themselves and live their own lives, we can nurture them, but we cannot make them like us. They are their own people, and we cannot impose ourselves onto them, they must live their own, authentic life.

They may see the world differently than we do, they will have their own feelings and experiences, wishes, and talents. They will spread their wings and create their own lives. This seems to be both our hope and sometimes our fear, as parents. These are lessons I try to carry with me every day.

Gibran talk about how, if anything, we should be inspired by our children and try to be more like them. That life goes only forwards, and they are our future. As parents, it's such a delicate balance. We want to guide our children with love and values, but also give them the freedom to explore and define who they are. We want to evolve ourselves, and always feel stable for our children.

Hilaria

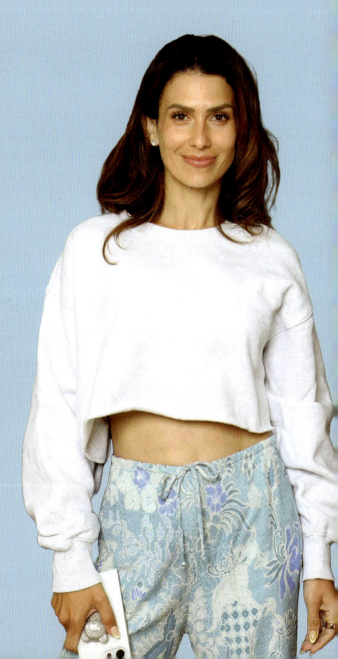

**On Children (1923)
by Kahlil Gibran**

And a woman who held a babe against her bosom said, Speak to us of Children.
And he said:
Your children are not your children.
They are the sons and daughters of Life's longing for itself.
They come through you but not from you,
And though they are with you yet they belong not to you.

You may give them your love but not your thoughts,
For they have their own thoughts.
You may house their bodies but not their souls,
For their souls dwell in the house of tomorrow, which you cannot visit, not even in your dreams.
You may strive to be like them, but seek not to make them like you.
For life goes not backward nor tarries with yesterday.
You are the bows from which your children as living arrows are sent forth.
The archer sees the mark upon the path of the infinite, and He bends you with His might that His arrows may go swift and far.
Let your bending in the archer's hand be for gladness;
For even as He loves the arrow that flies, so He loves also the bow that is stable.

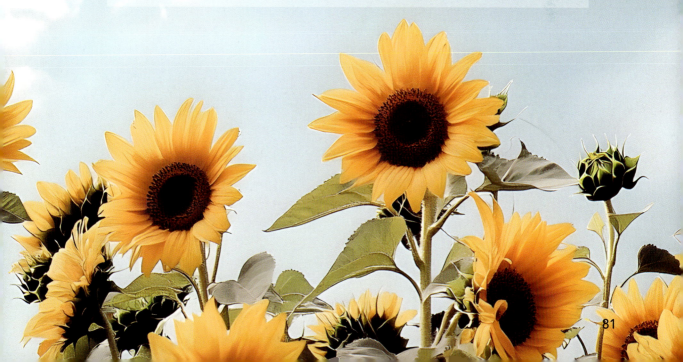

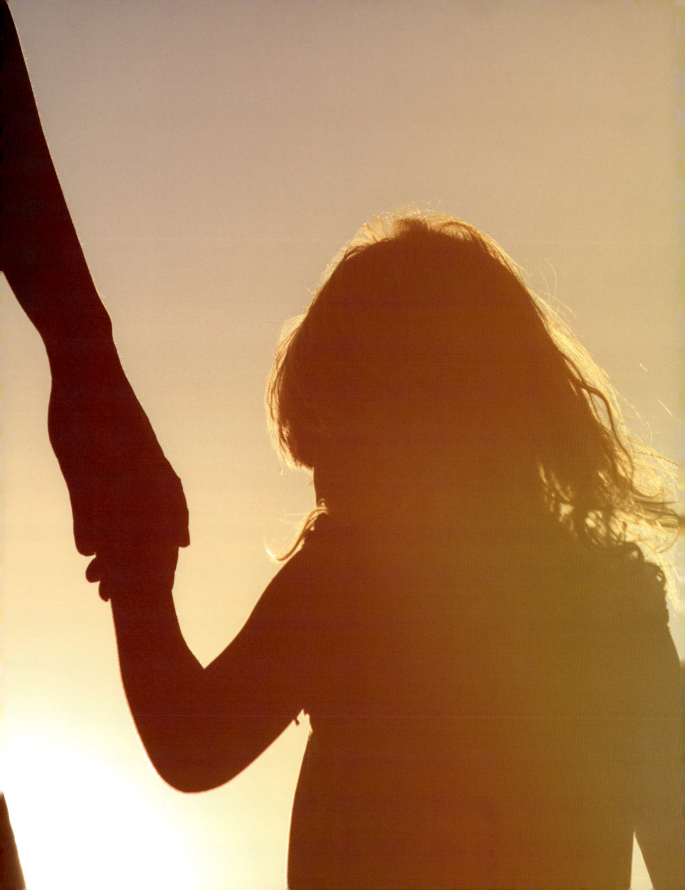

SAFE PLACE, SAFE SPACE

Not much in life comes with instructions these days — least of all children. And yet, here we are, navigating the ups and downs of raising these incredible, complicated humans, often without a clear map. Generations before us managed to raise families and keep society moving forward, and while that's comforting in theory, it doesn't make the day-to-day any easier.

We want our kids to have not just what they need, but hopefully what they want, too. We hope they'll do well in school, make friends, and avoid the sting of being left out or bullied. We want them to grow into kind, happy, healthy adults who can navigate the world responsibly and independently. We want them to have good, healthy boundaries and know how to stand up for themselves and others. We want to impossibly shield them from every heartache while encouraging them to be brave, curious, and resilient.

The world they are growing up in is not the same one that we knew as children. Technology is everywhere, and it never turns off. There's an endless stream of information — and fewer

tools for critical thinking. Our daughters are navigating girlhood in an environment that's faster, louder, and more judgmental than ever before.

It was intense when we were young, and now it's 24/7. By 10 or 11, so many girls are no longer wondering: what fun thing will I do today? Instead, they're asking themselves, How should I look today? They feel the unrelenting pressure to be "cool," to fit into a specific mold — whether that's about size, clothes, hair, or even how they pose in a photo.

The truth about raising daughters today is this: it takes equal parts patience and humor, a whole lot of love, and moments where you just hold on tight, praying the road smooths out soon. Our girls are growing up in a world that's dazzling and innovative but also overwhelming and judgmental. They're facing cultural pressures and temptations we couldn't have imagined at their age, and we're tasked with helping them make sense of it all.

More than ever, we moms need to be their safe place — a soft landing in a hard world. At the same time, we're responsible for setting boundaries and teaching them the values they'll carry with them for life. It's a balancing act like no other, but we show up every day because we believe in them. We believe in their strength, their potential, and their ability to grow into amazing women who will make this world better in ways we can't yet imagine.

For now, though? We're here, cheering them on, loving them hard, and hoping that, through it all, they never lose sight of who they are.

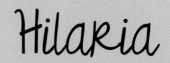

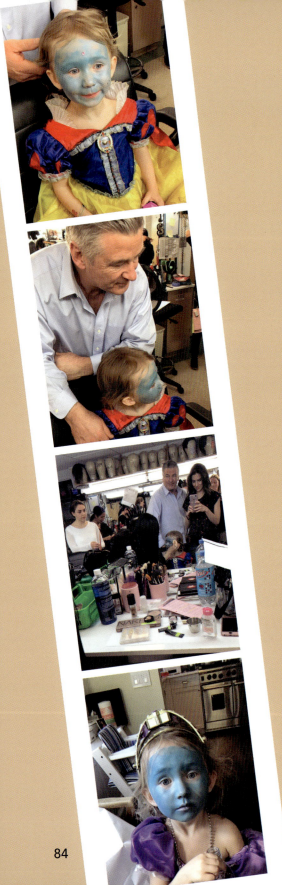

Carmen has always had such a vivid personality. Even as a toddler — not even three years old — her spark was impossible to miss. I'll never forget the day when she painted her whole face blue. Katy Perry had sent me her new lipstick line and one of the colors was bold, Smurf blue! Carmen, loving the color, began with her lips and then proceeded to color in her entire face! We were going to visit Alec on Saturday Night Live that evening, and she didn't want to take it off. I shrugged and went with it. We all had the most fun seeing this little kid, so confident with her self-expression. Until later, she had had enough, and thank goodness the SNL makeup pros were there to help us wipe it off! It was such a reflection of where she was at that time — so imaginative, so curious. So free. She loved to paint with acrylics, and she'd go all in. Our floors still carry little remnants of her colorful masterpieces from those years. Back then, she was drawn to the brightest, boldest colors. It was such a joy to watch her creativity blossom.

As Carmen grew older, her creativity evolved, as did her sense of self. She went through so many phases, each one part of her journey to figure out who she is. Her style changed constantly. At one point, she couldn't get enough of bold colors and fun dresses, and then, suddenly, dresses were out. She wanted nothing to do with anything flowy and instead opted for "pants and a shirt" every day. Now, like always, she is expressing herself through her style in ways that are self-driven and ever changing. There is no one right label to define her and I love this. As long as she is happy, I am happy.

That's the magic of childhood: discovering yourself through all these little shifts. As parents, it's such a delicate balance. We want to guide our children with love and values, but also give them the freedom to explore and define who they are. For us, it's about ensuring Carmen has a strong foundation while embracing and supporting each phase of her journey.

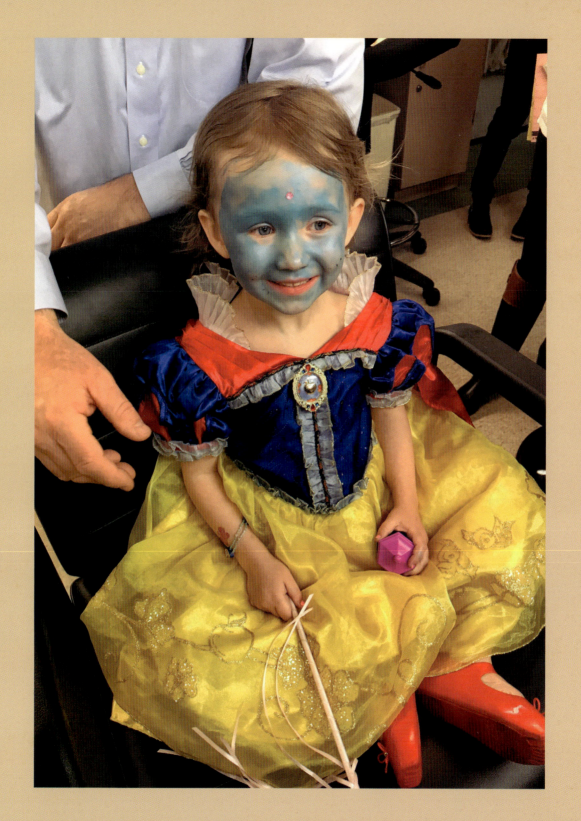

CREATIVITY IS QUEEN

Creativity is fun because you get to express yourself in ways that are authentic. Painting to doing makeup, acting, singing . . . there are so many unique ways to be creative. Everybody is different, and I feel the most like me when I'm doing something creative. It's like my brain quiets down, and I can just focus. I don't know exactly why I like creating things so much — I think it's about the process of creating, experimenting, and figuring things out along the way. It's just what makes me happy.

When I first got into skincare, I remember being completely fascinated by how different ingredients work together. It wasn't just about the final product; it was about learning something new and getting to use my hands to create. I started making my own face masks and sharing them with my mom, dad and siblings.

Maybe this creativity will help me figure out what I want to become? I try new things, and even if they don't stick, they teach me something about myself. It's how I've discovered what I like. From experimenting with makeup to learning how to bake with my siblings. Learning or creating with someone else is so fun. When you try something new with someone, you can laugh together when things go wrong and get excited together when things actually work. You can motivate each other, share tips, and figure it out together. Even when things don't go perfectly, it becomes a memory you can laugh about later.

Another thing I've learned is that creativity doesn't have to be successful to be worth it. Some of my favorite memories of creative projects are the ones where things didn't turn out quite how I expected. Like the time I tried to make a turmeric face mask with my mom. We tested it on my dad, and we ended up turning him orange! We couldn't stop laughing.

Creating is simply about having fun and enjoying the process and giving yourself permission to experiment, mess up, and try again. And doing this with friends and family is the best! I hope you find the same in your life!

Carmen

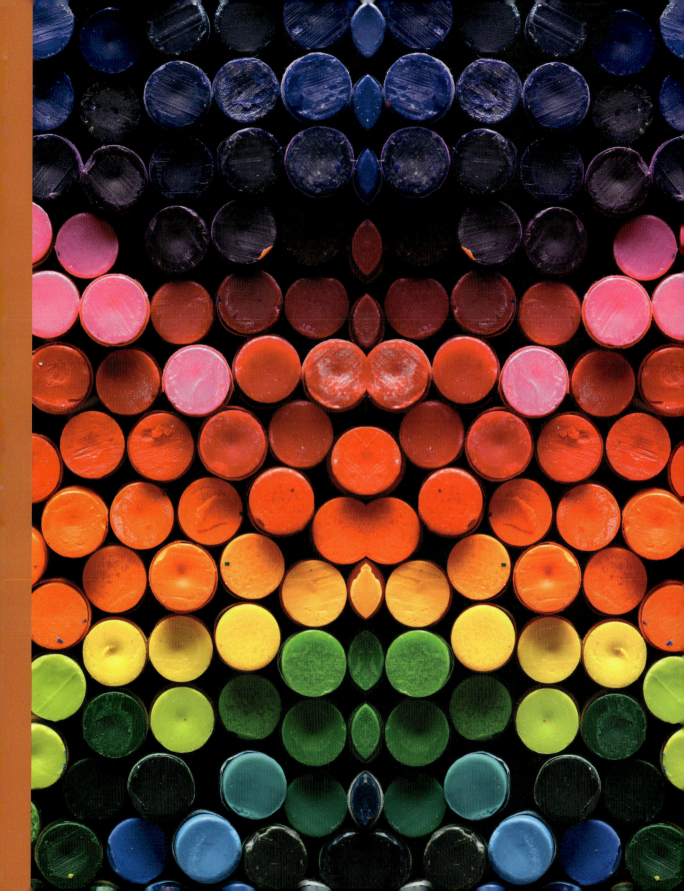

Sometimes Carmen will say things that are so wise beyond her years. One of the balances I try to do, as her mother, is to appreciate and foster her thoughts and advice, and sometimes calm her, by reminding her she can still be a kid. Every child has experiences where they exponentially grow and shift because of an unforeseen experience in life, good and bad. This is just part of being human. I really want to let her be a kid and have her know how valuable her thoughts are.

She's expressing herself and trying to connect with me, and that's such a beautiful thing. Listening to her has become a gift. She has this fresh perspective, and seeing the world through her eyes teaches me so much — not just about her, but about the world she's growing up in. I learn so much about myself and as a mother. It's humbling, really, and it reminds me how important it is to hear her. I encourage her to share her opinions openly.

In return, I share my own thoughts with her too. It's a two-way street. As Carmen grows, I want her to know she can always come to me — whether it's about her life, her worries, or even her thoughts about mine. I want her to feel my unwavering love, support, and honesty.

What I've come to realize is that our relationship is a partnership. Yes, I'm her mother, but we're also navigating life together. And in that partnership, there's so much room for growth, understanding, and connection.

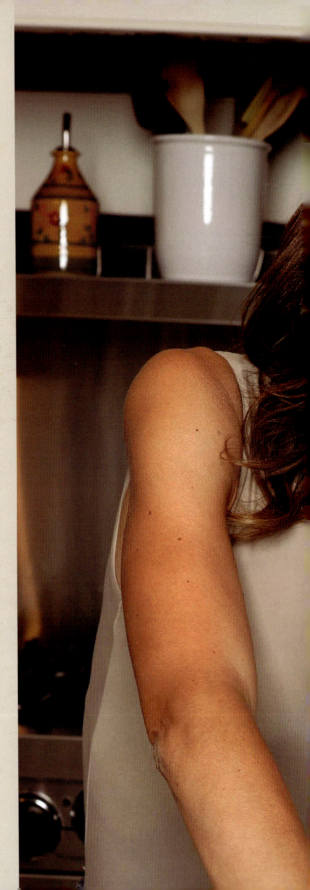

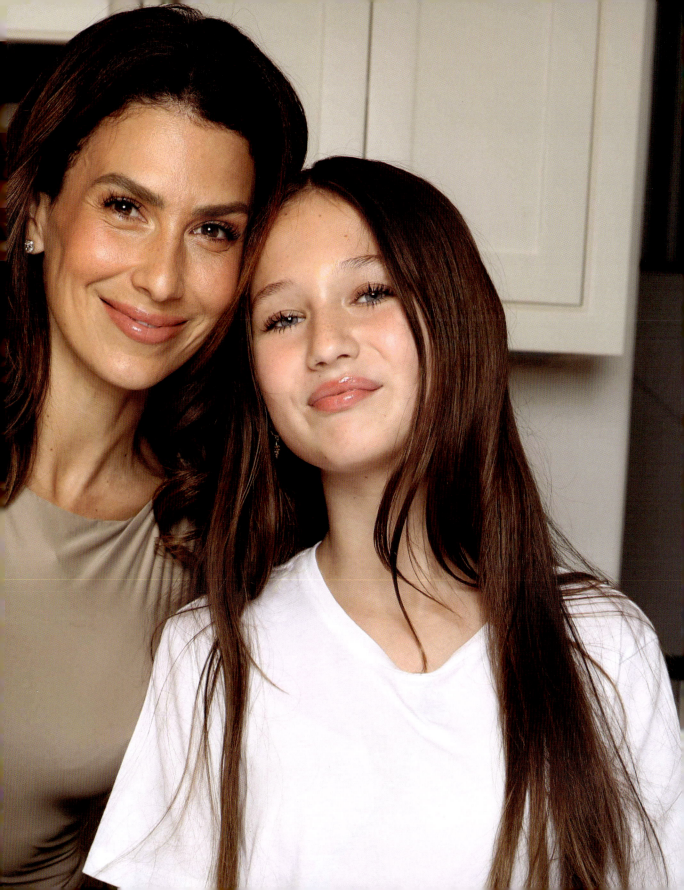

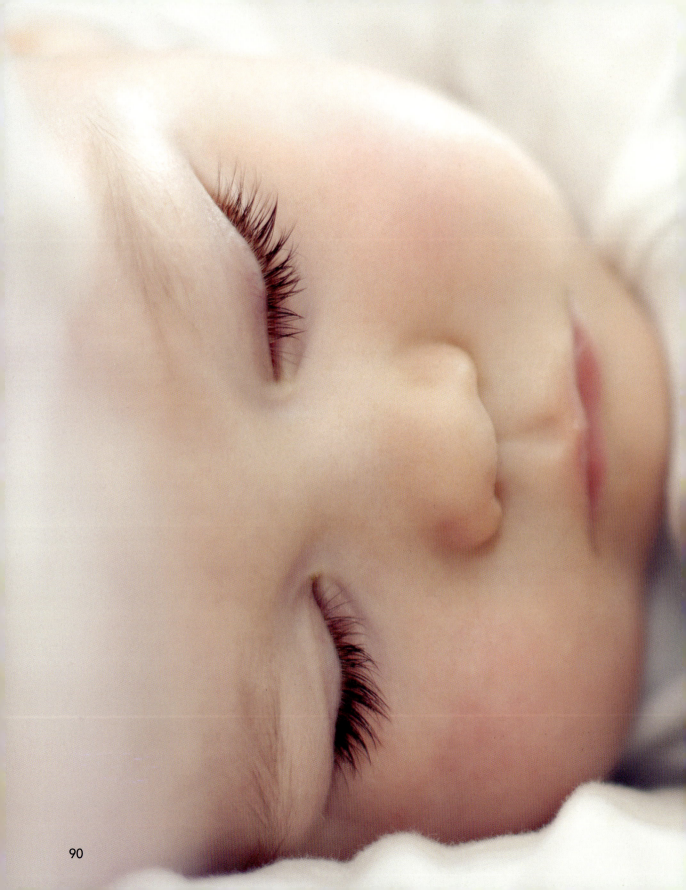

Carmen was my first baby, and, as a brand-new parent, I was so nervous about giving her anything. Even something as simple as Tylenol felt like such a big decision. Because there were no other babies in the house, she didn't get sick until she was eighteen months old. My other children had colds earlier because of their older, toddler siblings sharing and carrying home the germs they were getting at their preschool activities.

While I became more confident and less of my fearful, new parent former self, of course, we still paid close attention to every single thing we introduced into our children's systems. My kids laugh at me about how much I have relaxed and loosened up over the years and the many babies!

Parenting today can feel like such a mix of blessings and challenges. There's so much available to us now — and while that can be amazing, it can also be overwhelming.

I was a nervous first-time mother, but little by little, I learned to trust the process. I evolved by starting to let go.

Hilaria

CONNECTING WITH HER IS KEY

I don't know how you feel, but I think that building a strong, meaningful connection with our tween daughters might be one of the most rewarding aspects of parenting. These years are filled with significant transitions, both for her and for all of us. Amid the chaos of school schedules, social events, and extracurricular activities, there's an incredible opportunity to truly know them and be a part of their world. It's in these moments that we witness the spark of their unique personality — the quirks, talents, and dreams that make them who they are. Watching this individuality take shape is pure joy and a reminder of how incredible this journey of raising our daughters truly is.

Sharing in interests, no matter how different they might be from our own, is a simple but profound way to strengthen our bonds. Whether it's learning the lyrics to favorite songs, attending games, or diving into the latest trend they're obsessed with, our willingness to join in communicates that we value her passions. It's not necessarily about the activity itself — it's about showing that what matters to them matters to us. When they see that we're invested in their world, they feel seen and loved in ways that I can only imagine will strengthen our relationship.

It's important to acknowledge that these years of connection are fleeting. Our daughters won't stay little forever, and that's both a bittersweet reality and an incredible gift. Watching them grow into confident, competent young women is one of life's greatest privileges. While they still need our guidance, they're also learning to navigate the world in their own way. By staying close, we're not only helping them through the challenges of these phases, but we're also bearing witness to the amazing people they're becoming.

Meaningful connection obviously requires listening — not just to their words, but to what's behind them. Tweens often navigate complex emotions, and having a parent who listens without judgment can be a lifeline. When we make space for their feelings, no matter how big or small, we're teaching them that their voice matters and that they're worthy of being heard. This foundation of trust can empower them to approach the challenges of adolescence with greater confidence, knowing they have our unwavering support.

There's something magical about the shared laughter and inside jokes that develop when we're truly present in our children's lives. These small moments of joy create a reservoir of positivity that can strengthen our relationships during tougher times. Whether it's laughing over a silly meme they show us or dancing around the kitchen to their favorite playlist, these are the moments they will remember — times when they feel loved, cherished, and fully themselves.

Ultimately, connecting with our tween daughters is about showing them that they're deeply valued. It's about celebrating individuality while guiding with love and patience. As they grow, our relationships will evolve, but the effort we invest now lays the groundwork for a bond that will carry us through the years to come. These are the days when we get to truly know the incredible people our daughters are becoming, and that's a privilege worth cherishing.

Hilaria

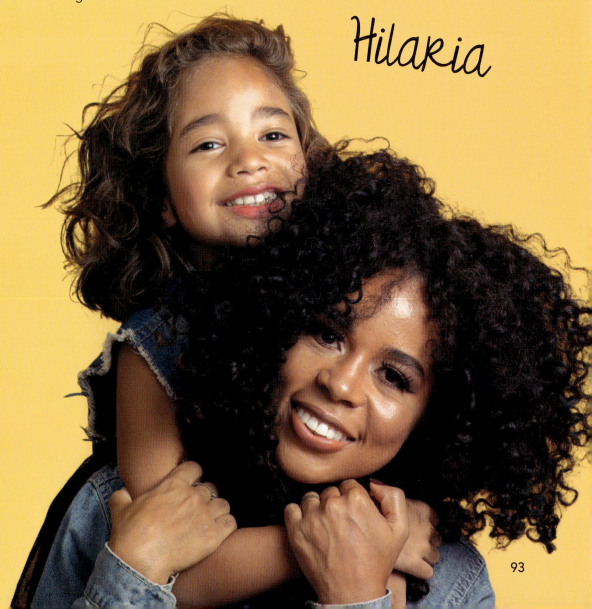

Hilaria

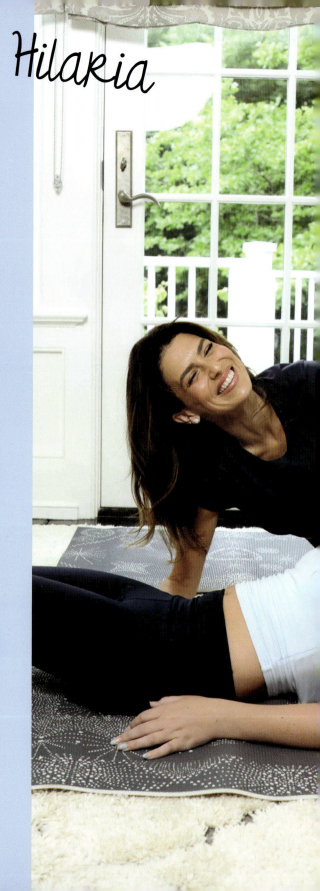

It is my value as a parent that I present myself in a way that allows each of my children to rely on me fully. Carmen tells me that she trusts me with everything. This is such a privilege. Hearing this means so much to me because it's a reflection of the time and effort I've poured into building a strong, close relationship with her — just as I do with each of my kids. Parenting is hard, and sometimes I wonder if I am getting things right or royally messing up. Probably a little bit…or sometimes a lot of bit…of both. But it is in these moments, when my children say such heartwarming things, that I feel like I am getting one or two things right! My goal is always to make them feel supported, safe, and deeply loved.

I've always believed in making each of my kids feel a little like an only child, even in the midst of our big family. What I mean by that is carving out individual quality time with each of them — time that's tailored to who they are and what they love. With one, it might be a walk through Central Park, with another, it could be window shopping, chatting about the things that catch their eye, playing a game, reading a book, or just being together and not doing anything in particular. Personalizing these moments makes them feel uniquely special, seen, and valued for who they are. It also allows me to enjoy each and every one of the children I feel privileged to mother.

Just like with my other children, Carmen and I don't need anything elaborate in order to connect. We can spend time doing something super simple, and it still feels so meaningful.

Instead of heading out for a new adventure, we often choose to stay home together, just the two of us. We love giving each other pedicures, painting our nails, or experimenting with different recipes in this book. One of our favorites is making lip scrubs — my go-to because it works so well. Carmen, of course, always has a new concoction or idea to try, and I adore seeing her creativity come to life.

These one-on-one moments mean so much to me. It's not just about the activity — it's about the time, the connection, and the love we share.

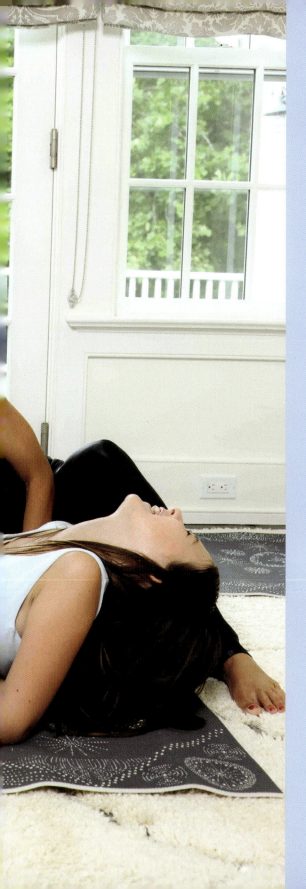

Spending time with my mom is one of my favorite things in the world. With a big family and so many siblings, having one-on-one time with her feels extra special. My absolute favorite tradition is our "date nights." Just the two of us — or sometimes we bring my dad, we spend the evening together and it means so much to me.. Sometimes we go to a restaurant we've been to before, where we always get the same order. Other times, we try new things. There are always new restaurants appearing in NYC. It doesn't matter where we go, though — it's the time we get to spend together that really makes it special.

I love how my mom spends time like this with each of us. She makes sure to do something that feels personal with each of my siblings, based on what they like. For me, we keep it simple and low-key, which is perfect.

My mom has always been a role model for me. She's so patient and generous with her time, and I always feel lucky to call her my mom. These date nights are a reminder of how much she cares, and I'll always treasure them.

Carmen

ACTIVITIES FOR MOM & DAUGHTER DUOS

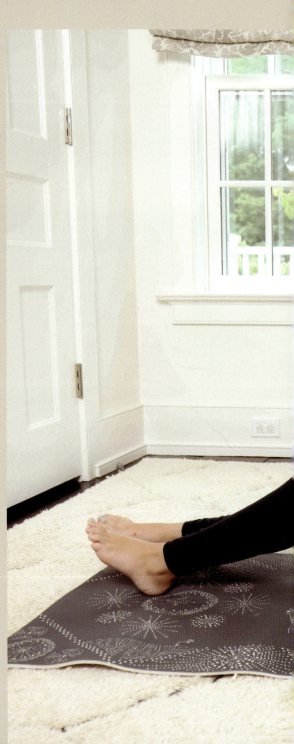

MOVE YOUR BODY:
Take a yoga class together
Go for a walk or run
Break out the bikes
Play your favorite sport
Hit the gym
Go to a climbing gym
Hike a local trail
Enjoy a beach day

SPARK THE SENSES:
Make a garden together
Paint each others nails
Try a new bubble tea shop
Go to formal afternoon tea
Share a spa day (at home is great!)
Watch a movie
Hunt for treasures at a local thrift store
Sing together at the top of your lungs

GET CREATIVE:
Visit a museum
Go to a concert
Have a retro living room dance party
Craft together
Attend a cooking class
Bake cookies or your favorite sweets
Take a painting or pottery class
Make jewelry, candles, or cosmetics
Learn something new together
Try a new recipe
Write your own recipe book!

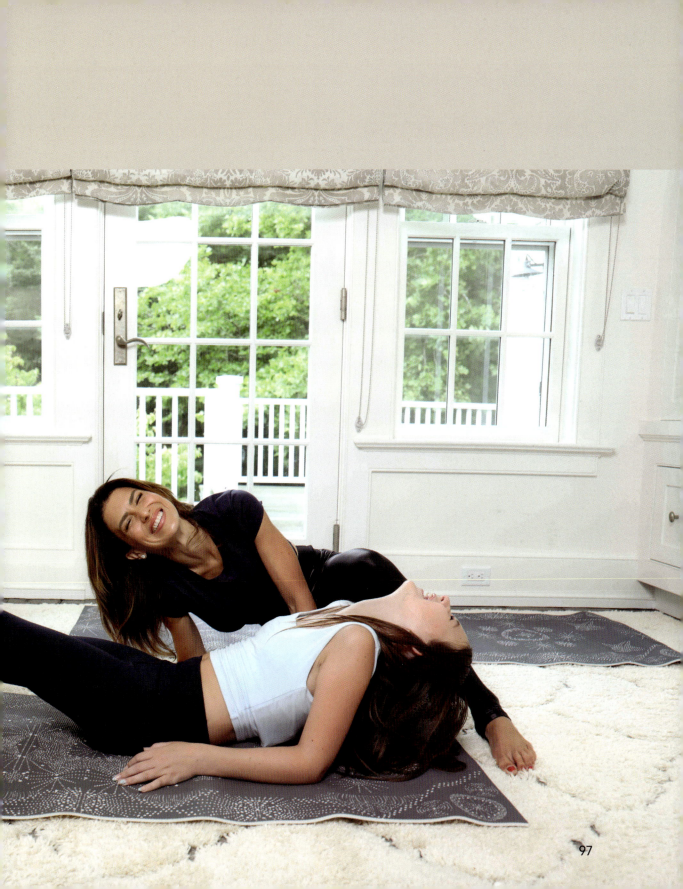

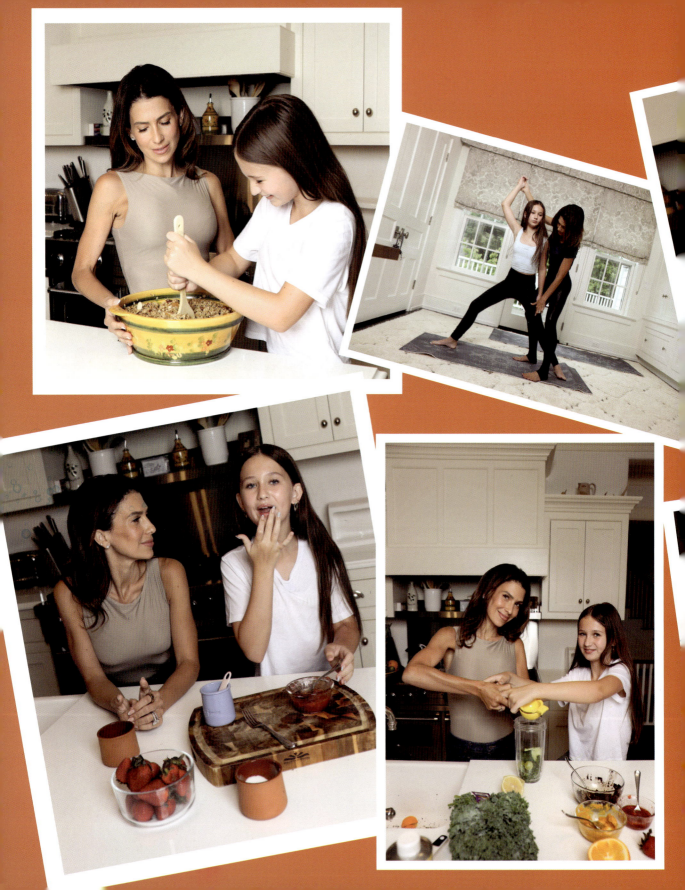

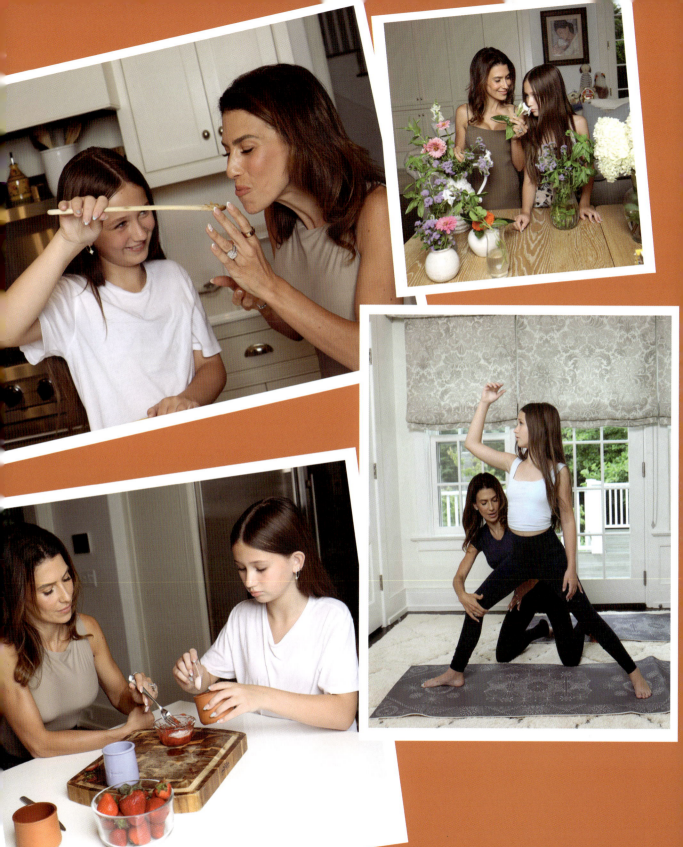

STAYING GROUNDED

In our house, we have lots of animals and people! I love how full our home is and that there is always something fun happening, but I also really like spending time alone. I've learned how to tune out the noise of our loud home.

When I need alone time, I often grab bowls and ingredients from the kitchen and close myself off in the bathroom and mix and create. I love to listen to music, pamper myself, chat with my friends, and just be by myself.

I am a big sister and I help my parents out a lot in the house and with our family. I love being those things, and my mom tells me that I need to also just be me. She talks a lot about yoga and mindfulness and I am not sure I always understand what she is saying, but I think I get the closest when I am taking my "me time," as she tells me is important.

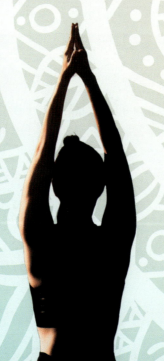

YOGA

My siblings and I always love doing yoga with my mom. I mean . . . how cool is it that she can do headstands and handstands and put her legs behind her head?! We will all get together in our living room and have so much fun, trying new poses and tricks. She has always taught us to focus on our breath and our hearts and, in hard moments, to pay attention to them. She teaches us breathing exercising that can slow down our heart, when we are upset. So we learn that yoga isn't just fun poses, it also can make us feel better.

MEDITATION

I have been to my mom's yoga classes, and she says that sometimes meditation can be overwhelming when you are just beginning. It's because to tell someone to just immediately clear their minds and think of nothing feels impossible! She tells us that our minds are busy and are built to think and want to focus on things. She tells the class and us at home that if we focus our minds on our bodies and our breath, we can calm them. That this is an important step in meditation. So when we are upset, she has us lay down with one hand on our heart and one on our belly, and we breathe and make our mind focus on our heartbeat and breath. We try to make our breaths longer and our hearts slower. If we keep our mind focused on this task, we find that we calm our mind. When we feel better, we can solve our problems better and together.

MINDSET

We talk a lot about gratitude in our family, so I have learned to focus on what I am thankful for. When I feel really down or upset, reminding myself of how many things are going right helps so much. It doesn't mean that I am not still upset about whatever is going on, it just means that I can also be happy for good things. This happy makes the sad seem not as overwhelming.

I also express what's stressing me out, or anything else taking up a lot of space in my mind. It's a release of negative energy. I always talk to my mom about what is bothering me too — this helps so much.

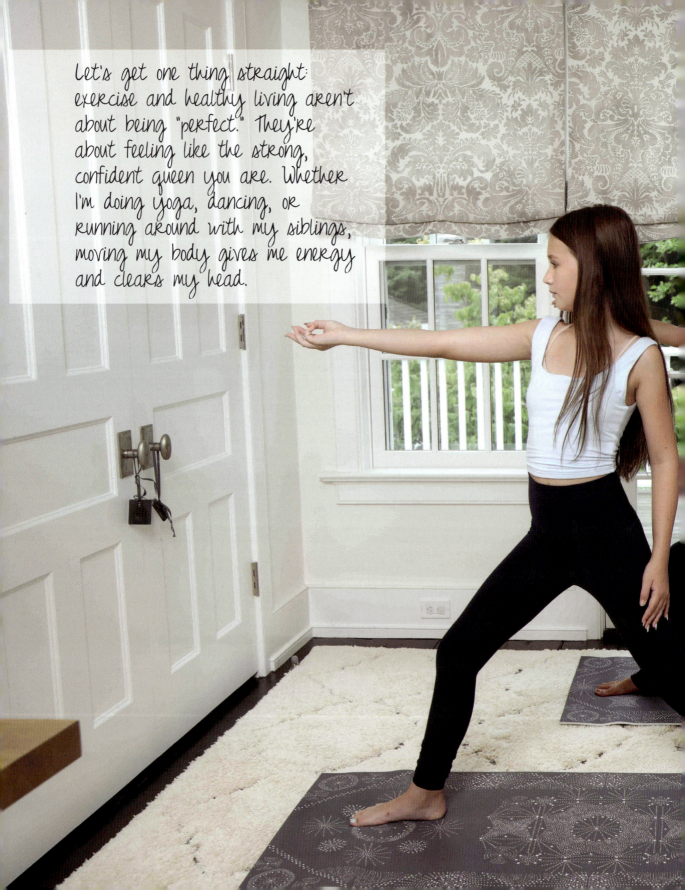

Let's get one thing straight: exercise and healthy living aren't about being "perfect." They're about feeling like the strong, confident queen you are. Whether I'm doing yoga, dancing, or running around with my siblings, moving my body gives me energy and clears my head.

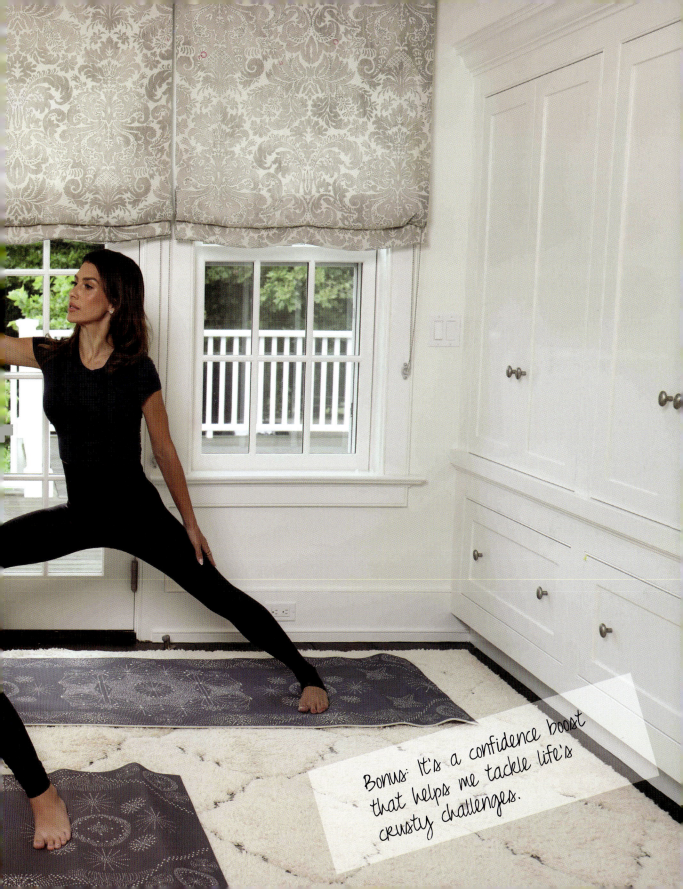

Bonus: It's a confidence boost that helps me tackle life's crusty challenges.

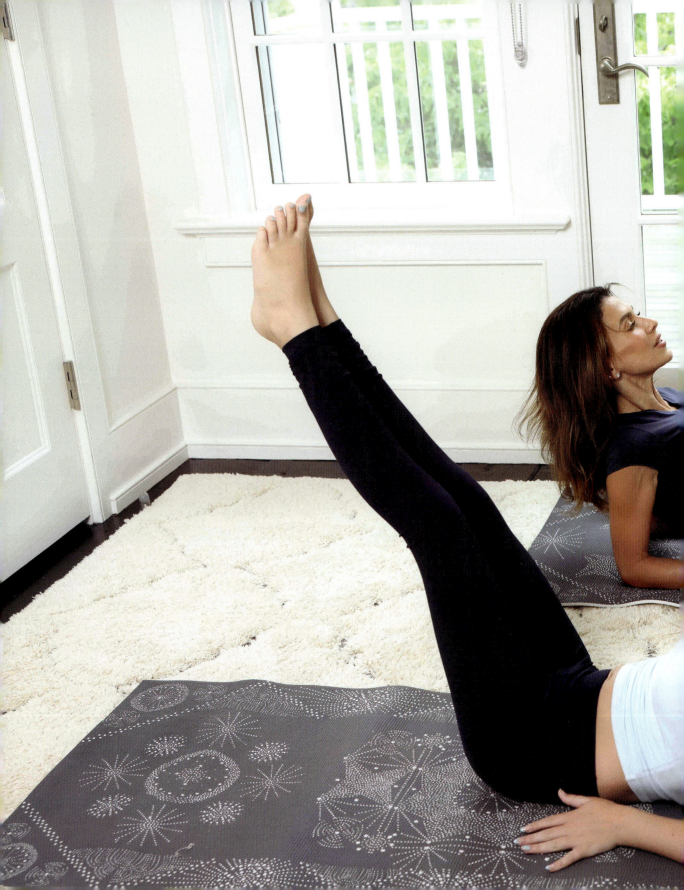

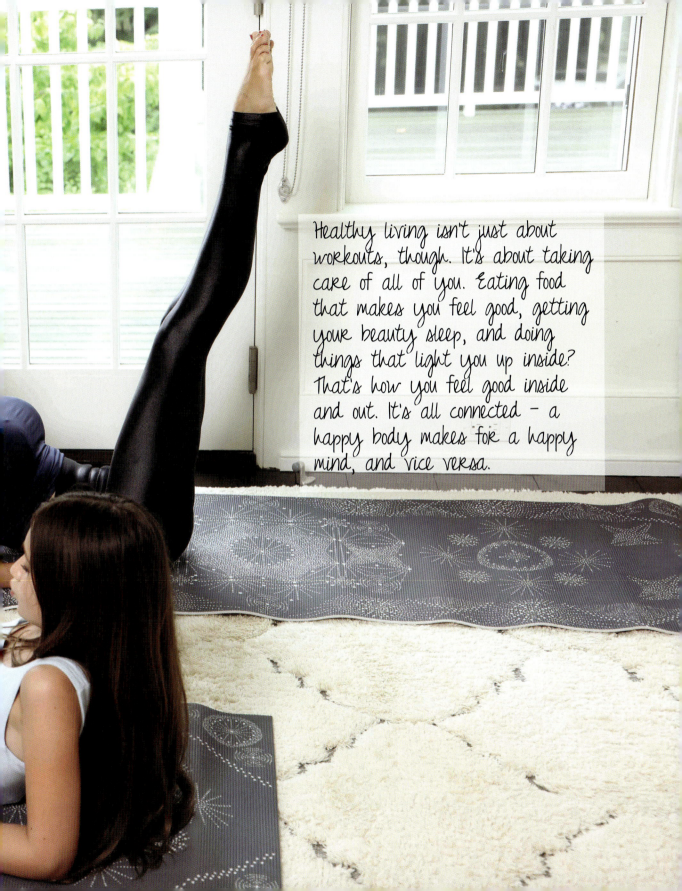

Healthy living isn't just about workouts, though. It's about taking care of all of you. Eating food that makes you feel good, getting your beauty sleep, and doing things that light you up inside? That's how you feel good inside and out. It's all connected — a happy body makes for a happy mind, and vice versa.

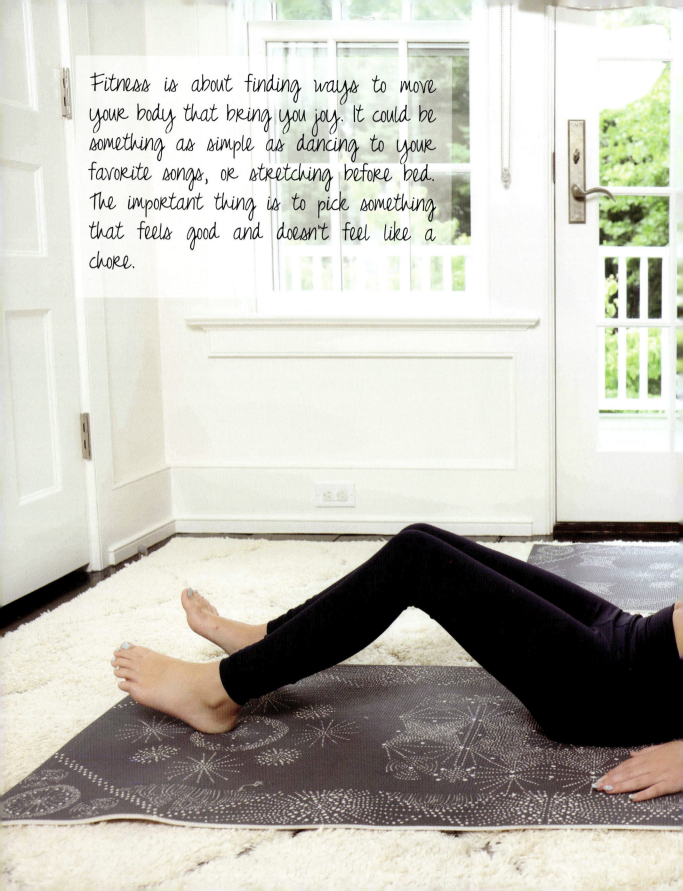

Fitness is about finding ways to move your body that bring you joy. It could be something as simple as dancing to your favorite songs, or stretching before bed. The important thing is to pick something that feels good and doesn't feel like a chore.

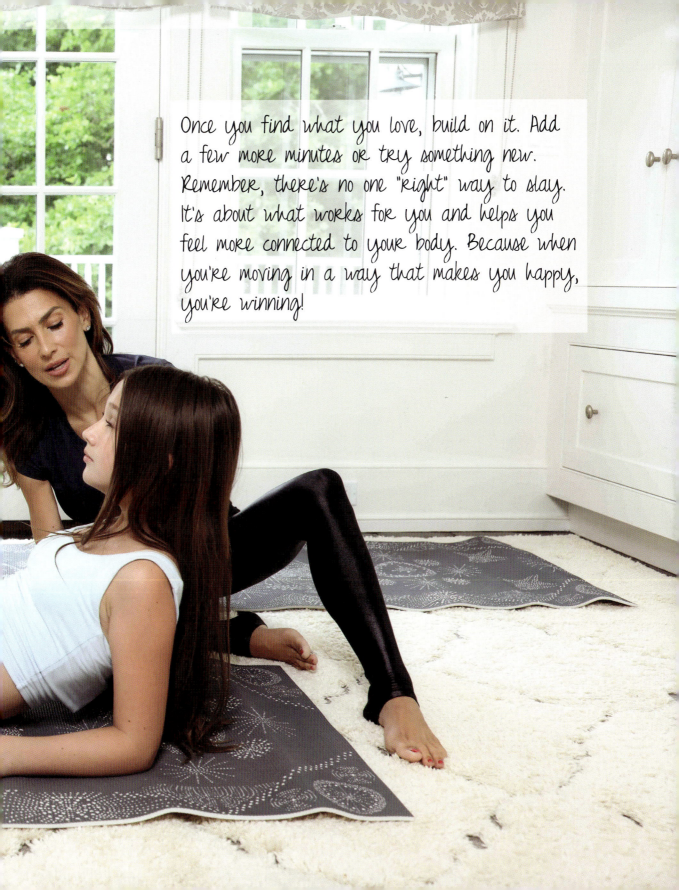

Once you find what you love, build on it. Add a few more minutes or try something new. Remember, there's no one "right" way to slay. It's about what works for you and helps you feel more connected to your body. Because when you're moving in a way that makes you happy, you're winning!

MOM TESTED,

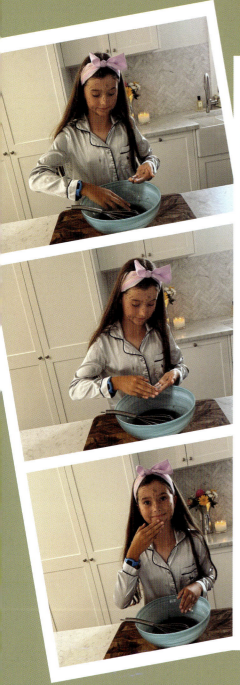
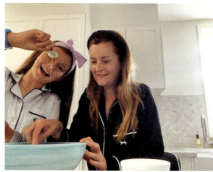
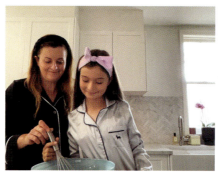
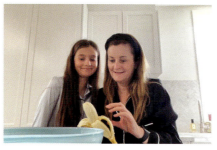
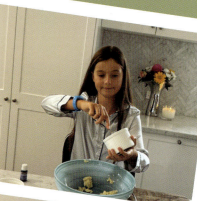
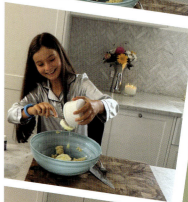
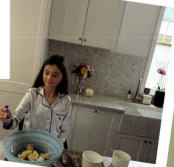

Ros and Olivia (11) testing Glow Getter Chia Mask, Sweet Slumber Night Time Mask, and Shiny Hair, I Care Mask

MOM APPROVED

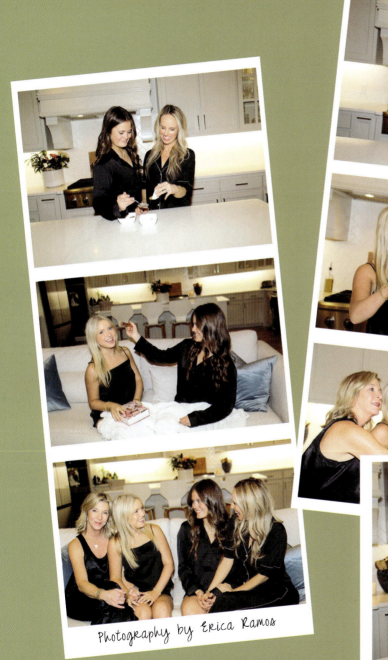
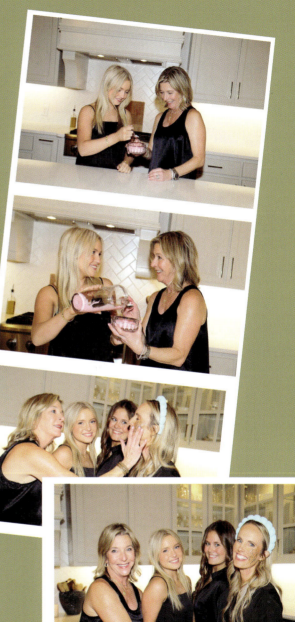

Photography by Erica Ramos

Lindsay and Allie-Gwyn (15) and Kyndal and Abby (14) test Glow Getter Chia Mask and Silky Smooth Body Scrub

CELEBRATING MOM & ME

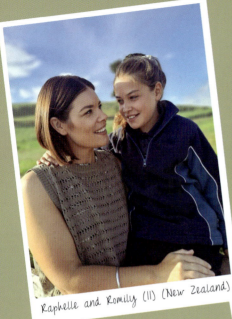

Raphelle and Romilly (11) (New Zealand)

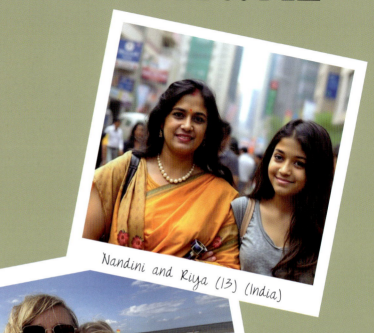

Nandini and Riya (13) (India)

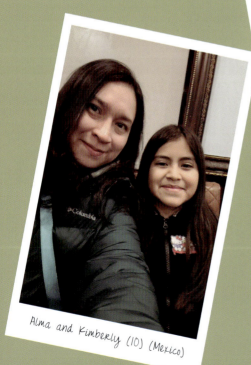

Alma and Kimberly (10) (Mexico)

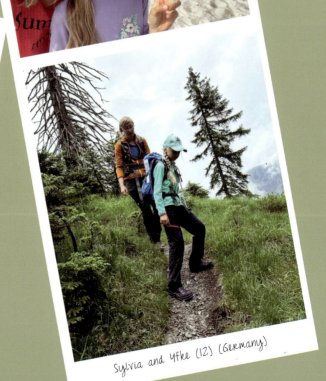

Sylvia and Yfke (12) (Germany)

AROUND THE WORLD

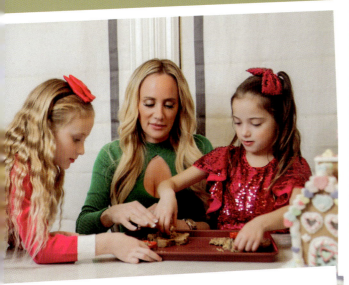

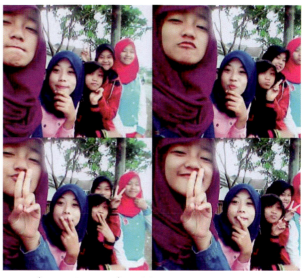

Eka and Arysky (10) Liia, Sri (9) and Sundri (11) (Indonesia)

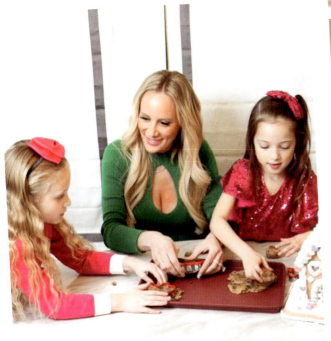

Erica, Aspen (6), and Holland (8) (USA)

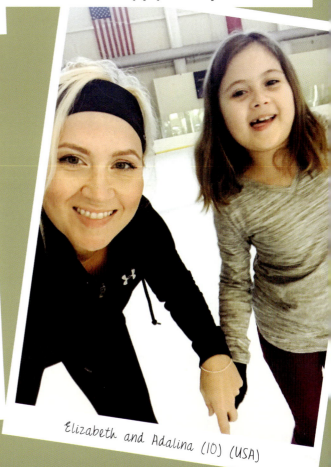

Elizabeth and Adalina (10) (USA)

NOTE FROM THE PUBLISHER

At DAP, we believe in the power of connection, tradition, and the simple joys of shared experiences. That's why we're so excited to bring you this book, a celebration of natural beauty, skincare, and self-care rituals passed between mothers and daughters. In today's fast-paced world, the moments we share with our loved ones — especially those that nurture both our bodies and our spirits — are more important than ever.

This book is more than a guide; it's an invitation. It invites mothers and daughters to explore the beauty of self-care together — a time-honored tradition from around the world, and a chance to create their own rituals that honor their unique bond. Teaching young women about self-care isn't just about skincare routines or beauty tips — it's about instilling confidence, fostering mindfulness, and nurturing a sense of self-worth that will serve them throughout their lives.

I founded DAP to bring powerful stories to the world, and what's more powerful than a connection between a mother and her daughter? Through the experience of working on this book with Hilaria and Carmen, we have seen firsthand the love, patience, and encouragement that this mother shows to her daughter. In a time where TikTok takes the attention of so many young girls, it is encouraging to see pure moments of connection shared from the material bond.

This book's thoughtfully curated recipes, tips, and activities are not only easy to follow but also celebrate the natural world and its incredible power to heal and restore. Whether it's blending a soothing face mask in the kitchen, learning the benefits of simple ingredients, or sharing a quiet moment together, this book is a tool for building connection and empowerment.

Our hope is that this book becomes a cherished resource for mothers and daughters — a source of inspiration, laughter, and love. May it remind you to celebrate your inner and outer beauty, and to find joy in the little moments that bring you closer together.

Thank you to Hilaria and Carmen for letting us be a part of your journey.

Sequoia, and the DAP Team

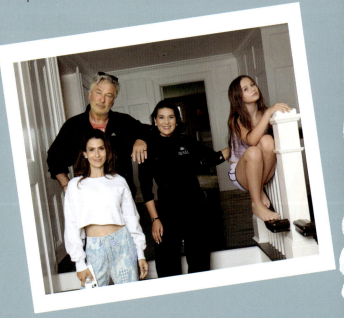

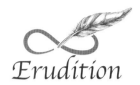

ABOUT THE PUBLISHER

Di Angelo Publications was founded in 2008 by Sequoia Schmidt—at the age of seventeen. The modernized publishing firm's creative headquarters is based in Los Angeles. In 2020, Di Angelo Publications made a conscious decision to move all printing and production for domestic distribution of its books to the United States. The firm is comprised of ten imprints, and the featured imprint, Erudition, was inspired by the desire to spread knowledge, spark curiosity, and add numbers to the ranks of continuing learners, big and small.

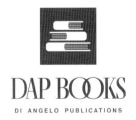